Shared Reading

Jan Raes

The Ultimate Therapy

Lannoo Campus

Contents

Prologue 8

A simple methodology that makes great things possible 14
A cyclical dynamic of change in five phases 16
The freedom to be, without labels and medical files 18
The first steps 19

1 **Starting** 22

Breaking through patterns of habit 25
Inspired to take action 28
Dealing safely with the unpredictable 33
Tips for practice 35

2 **Growing** 36

Growing: a multi-dimensional process 38
Shared Reading as a free space for growth 40
   The story as a zone of experience 42
      The conversation space during the breaks in the reading 44
         Mirror neurons 44

Expanding the mental-emotional space 50
   In education, care & support, and therapy 52
   In Shared Reading 54
The therapeutic power of Shared Reading 56
   Imagination 56
   Beyond the pain point 57
   Flexible distance for difficult themes 59
   Embracing the shadow side and unreachable experiences 61
An associative process 63
Tips for practice 65

3 Harvesting 68

A time to harvest: gathering what you have rightly earned 69
The harvest of Shared Reading 72
   Increased possibilities 72
   Seeing the universal in the personal 74
   Safety 78
      Transfer: the reading companion as a parent figure 80
   Strength 85
   Building blocks for a caring society 87
      Powerful therapeutic effects without high costs 90
The necessary conditions for harvesting 91
   Slowness and serenity 91
   Giving the participants the freedom they need 96
Tips for practice 99

4 **Learning** 100

   Sifting and letting go 102
   Clearing the clutter from your mind 104
   Letting go and keeping hold of fragments: dementia 107
   Shared mental-emotional space as a learning space 111
   Neuroplasticity: flexible brains 112
   No obligation to learn 117
   Letting go of rigidity in care organisations 121
   Tips for practice 126

5 **Relaxing** 128

   Re-energising the depths of your being 130
   A society in overdrive 132
      Burnout 135
   Shared Reading as a process of deepening 136
   Taking people seriously 142
   Tips for practice 144

Epilogue 146

   The cycle of healing and integration 151
      Het Lezerscollectief 152
      Starting with Shared Reading? 153
   Sources for the literary fragments 155

Prologue

I was repairing a flat tyre on my bike and had just sworn at the fifth patch I had failed to place properly, when the telephone rang.

– He has fallen over. It's probably nothing serious. But perhaps it's best if you come and have a look?

Grumbling at this unnecessarily exaggerated female sense of concern, I rushed over to the playground where I had ditched my son for the holidays, so that I could enjoy a bit of peace and quiet.

She walked towards me, holding the boy by his hand. The universe came to a halt. I was deaf. I was dumb. My soul shrivelled in ecstasy.

A quarter of an hour later, I went home, dragging along Pieter-Jan like some kind of excess baggage, with him no doubt planning to find a lover for my wife who would be more reliable than myself.

On the way, I bought a new tyre for the bike. Having fixed it to the wheel, I locked myself away and wrote a poem.

Out of this poem, a strategy gradually emerged.

All day and half the night I sat in my room, mumbling, muttering but stubbornly proving my point. I was proving that she was the most beautiful woman in the world, that she loved me, that God existed and that our love was His will. I was proving that she got up during the night to be melancholy, reducing her diary to no more than thoughts of me and stretching out her hands in the mirror towards mine. After ten whiskies, I finally proved that her tears would one day wet my grave and that her fame for later generations would be assured. And all this I did in no more than twelve quatrains, so that the power of proof in each line was overwhelming.

Fragment from: Charles Ducal, 'Judith'

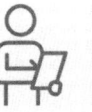 In the building where my office is located a session of Shared Reading[1] was organised for a group of people who were interested. I had already heard something about it – people coming together to listen to stories read aloud and then discussing them – but I was still sketchy about the details. In the corridor I bumped into my friend Dirk. He invited me to come along to the session. 'Who knows, perhaps it's something for you, Jan,' he said. 'So why not pop in, if you've got the time. Then you'll know!' I am curious by nature and I did have a bit of free time, so I thought: 'Why not?'

When I walked into the room, I saw nine people sitting in comfortable chairs. On the table in the middle there were tea and biscuits. It looked relaxed, like it might be fun. I joined the circle and after a brief introduction the woman leading the session explained what text we would be shared reading.

Everyone opened a book that they had been given before the session began. 'Great,' I thought, 'now I'm sitting here like a right idiot. Why on earth did I agree to come? It's not as though I haven't got lots of other things to do!' A little voice inside my head told me to stop moaning and make the most of it. And so I decided to just

---

1 In this book I use the term Shared Reading to refer to the specific methodology used by Het Lezerscollectief, based on the Shared Reading methodology developed by Jane Davis for the British organisation The Reader.

listen to the text and see what, if anything, it did for me. After all, I was here now, wasn't I? The least I could do was to play my part.

It was a nice text, about a father doing some odd jobs at home. I'm a bit of an odd-job man myself, so I soon found myself getting into the swing of things. To my surprise, I discovered that I felt calm and relaxed in this new setting, reading along with someone who is used to reading out loud at a gentle pace. It made me think of my teacher in the fifth form at secondary school, who used to read in this same pleasant way on Fridays after the mid-afternoon break, provided we had been good. I was starting to enjoy the simple act of listening. All thoughts about work and its associated pressures had disappeared and I immersed myself in the emotions of the main character.

Oh dear! Suddenly he falls madly in love with his son's teacher! He needs to pick up the lad from the playground where he has fallen over and the moment he sees her... Bam! Head over heels! He is no longer interested in his son. All he is concerned about is his own exaggerated feelings. In my mind's eye, I can see it happening! What a plonker!

The rest of the text continues to explore his infatuation and his behaviour, fictional though it is, starts to irritate me. A whole string of none-too-complimentary comments flash through my brain. *'What on earth does the idiot think he is doing? Is he planning to just dump his wife? Instead of trying to come to terms with the situation, he immediately wants to find a radical solution to satisfy his own emotions. My God, this man has some really aggressive fantasies!'*

I realise that the main character is making me angry and am surprised that the story has such a powerful and lifelike impact on my imagination. Funny, I thought that only happened when you were reading to yourself, but the sensation seems to be even stronger with reading aloud.

There is a short break. 'And?' asks the woman leading the session. 'What are your first impressions?'

'Romantic,' says a woman with greying hair. 'It reminds me of my own youth.'

'Wonderful,' adds a man. 'That feeling of butterflies in your stomach: there's nothing like it.'

I remain silent, but think: *'So they both go along with his infatuation, as though there is nothing wrong with it. But what about the wife? Just trade her in like a used car? A new model to replace the old one? No, that's not on!*

It suddenly strikes me that *my* reading of the story is not the only possible reading, and that the interpretations of the other participants are both surprisingly interesting and valid. By listening to what they have to say, a number of doors open inside my head, each leading to alternative paths for the continuation and completion of the story. Yes, this first meeting with my fellow readers has been an interesting one. Or should I say my fellow travellers in our literary love bubble? I find it admirable that they are so willing to throw themselves into this emotional maelstrom!

During the first round of questioning and discussion, I hold my peace. Slightly worried, I ask myself whether or not I am so quick to make black-and-white judgements in daily life. The others in the group seem milder and more forgiving. Next to me sits a teacher, who is clearly enjoying herself. Opposite there is a pensioner, who says that precisely the same thing happens to him whenever he falls in love, although it no longer happens as often as it used to! *'Hm,'* I think, *'perhaps that's something to think about after the session.'* 'I'm curious to find out how it all ends,' says another man. 'He is so passionate, anything could happen.'

The story continues, steadily going from bad to worse. The man convinces himself with each new whisky that he is truly in love and that she, impassioned by his romantic verses, will one day melt in his arms. No doubt about it... But that's not how I

> see it. This can only end in disaster... 'Fun, isn't it,' says someone next to me during the next break. I nod affirmatively. But it's actually more than just fun, it's wonderful...

After this first introduction to Shared Reading, I was fascinated by the concept. It all seemed so simple: people meet to listen to or to read along with a literary text, pausing every now and then to discuss the contents. You can't get much simpler than that, can you?

Yet simple or not, it is super-effective. The more testimonies I heard from people who regularly took part in the reading sessions, the more I realised that this kind of interaction focused on literary texts had made a real impact on them. I heard stories of people who rediscovered their courage during the sessions, saw the first glimmer of light at the end of the long tunnel of their depression, found something to hold on to, notwithstanding the difficult circumstances in their private and/or professional lives. They made a point of faithfully attending every reading group, no matter what else was noted in their diaries and busy agendas. Even people who never said a word during the discussion moments explained to me that the sessions were important to them: 'It is just being at the meetings that counts,' said one regular participant.

Impressed by these testimonies, I decided to put my shoulder behind the praiseworthy efforts of Het Lezerscollectief, a network of people who organise and conduct Shared Reading sessions throughout Flanders. This makes it possible for people who have little or no access to literature to experience the transforming effect of powerful stories and poems.

A simple methodology that makes great things possible

At first glance, the methodology of Shared Reading is very simple: people meet on a regular basis (for example, every week or every fortnight), either in a reading group or individually with a reading companion. This companion, who is a member of the Lezerscollectief team, chooses an ambiguous literary text in advance and reads it aloud to the group or the reading partner. In a single session it is usual to read a short story and a poem. The participants are given a copy of the texts, so that they can follow them silently while they are being read. At certain moments agreed in advance the companion will stop reading and ask a number of questions about the texts and their contents. The focus is placed primarily on the thoughts, associations and feelings that the texts arouse in the participants, so that an authentic conversation can be developed. After this period of expression and/or dialogue, the companion resumes reading. Within this simple format, the most remarkable things can happen; things that are powerful or subtle, therapeutic, liberating, heart-warming, etc. – but only if the process is approached with a sufficient degree of care and nuance.

In practice, Shared Reading usually takes place in a group rather than an individual context. Twelve participants and a single reading companion is the maximum number for this process to be comfortable and effective. Eight participants and a companion is ideal, but smaller groups are also possible. The advantage of the group is that it promotes a wider range of interaction, so that a greater number of different insights and perspectives are raised, which enhances the growth and learning processes of those taking part.

Reading aloud to just a single person is possible, but more difficult. It demands greater attention and a more specific approach from the companion to sense what is going on inside the listener. It is also necessary for the personalities of companion and reader to click, so that sufficient trust and openness can be generated to make possible a deep and meaningful conversation. In a duo, the companion plays a more active role in the conversation, since this is the best way to help the listener to view the story from different perspectives. Within this conversation, it is important for the companion to find the right balance between making his/her own suggestions and drawing suggestions from the listener. The advantage of a reading duo is that all the attention is focused on the listener, so that he/she can benefit from a personal experience rather than a shared experience with others.

Shared Reading seeks to reach, among others, people who are vulnerable: persons with physical or mental difficulties or limitations, those living in poverty, those confined to prison, etc. People in these categories do not always have access to thought-provoking literature or else their social background often leads them to be categorised as 'people who are not interested in books'.

But practice has shown that nothing could be further from the truth! People who read or listen to powerful literature and then discuss it not only experience connection with others and a deepening of their own thoughts, but also come to see new possibilities in their lives and achieve a level of calm that allows them to make well-considered decisions. They integrate new insights into their thinking and learn to let go of the things they no longer need. By exchanging reactions and experiences with others they realise that their own perspective is not the only perspective and that other views on reality – and on their own life – are possible. The Shared Reading process, especially if it is regularly repeated in a series of reading sessions, opens the door to a whole range of unexpected sensations and emotions that can have a deeply healing effect on people, irrespective of whatever literary baggage they might carry.

A cyclical dynamic of change in five phases

Shared Reading initiates a process of change in people that operates in accordance with a universal pattern. It is possible to observe the same dynamic in many aspects of our world: in nature, in our personal development as human beings, in companies and organisations, etc. This process is cyclical and takes place in different phases.

1. Every change begins with a **start phase**, in which people take the initiative and seek to make something happen. This is the phase of dynamism and action.
2. The energy of this initial burst of activity **grows** and expands, so that old habits and limiting patterns of thought are pushed aside. This growth creates more room for people's true thoughts and emotions, so that their thinking and feeling becomes freer and more flexible.
3. When the growth phase has passed its zenith, the moment has arrived for **harvesting**: people fully integrate the insights they have acquired during the growth phase into their being. This gives them new strength.
4. Deeper understanding and greater strength initiates a new phase of **learning**: through a process of slow and careful introspection people become able to distinguish which parts of their inner harvest they wish to retain and which parts they wish to let go.
5. By letting go of the things they no longer need, people are able to achieve a true sense of **ease**. This is the phase of calm, which allows people to glean even deeper insights. This relaxed process of reflection generates new reserves of inspiration and willpower, which makes it possible to start with new initiatives – and so the circle is completed and the cycle can begin again, but now at a higher level.

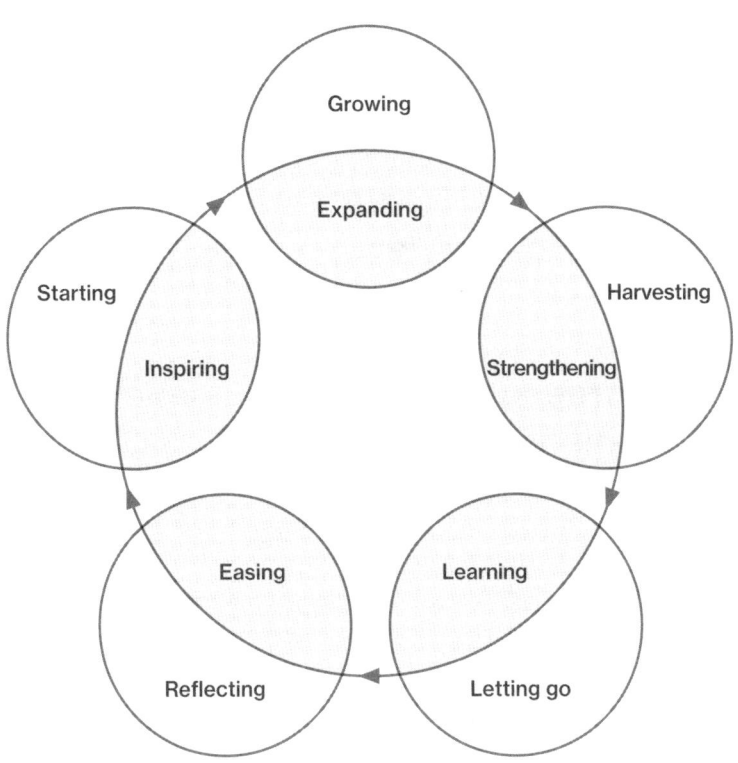

The five phases of change

In this book I will sketch how this dynamic unfolded in five phases in Shared Reading, with examples and testimonies from the field of health care.[2] In passing, I will also highlight the differences and similarities between the Shared Reading methodology and traditional forms of therapy and care. At the end of each chapter you will find a series of tips that will help you to initiate the process in your own work context, via reading groups or reading duos.

The freedom to be, without labels or a medical file

Given my background as a doctor and psychiatrist, I was particularly interested in what Shared Reading might mean for the care sector. As it turned out, quite a lot! The procedure has now been applied successfully in a number of different care contexts: in residential homes for the elderly (both for the mentally healthy and for those who are in the early stages of dementia); special youth rehabilitation centres; psychiatric hospitals; centres for mental health care; recovery academies; care centres for people with a mental or physical limitation; ordinary hospitals.

Shared Reading sets in motion something that does people good. In a sector that is overflowing with procedures, structures and organisational and therapeutic objectives, it creates a free space for the patient or client; a place where all the clinical labels can be forgotten and where no one has the person's medical file in the back of their mind or assesses them in terms of progress, healing or recovery. In this space, there is only one thing that counts: the freedom to listen, the freedom to read along with the text and, if you so desire, the freedom to discuss its contents.

---

[2] The names of the people in the examples and testimonies have been changed to protect their privacy.

Because even this latter aspect is by no means obligatory: if you just want to sit there and listen in silence, you are free to do so.

This freedom is like a breath of fresh air for the patient or client. He or she does not have to do anything, but has the option to actually do quite a bit, if that is what he or she wants. And that can generate unexpected but unmistakeably healing effects. In short, Shared Reading often works better than pills and therapy. And that is the story that I would like to tell in the following five chapters.

The first steps

Do you want to discover for yourself what Shared Reading can do for you, so that perhaps later you can apply its methodology in your field of work? You do? In that case, you are about to embark on a fascinating voyage of exploration. The best way to learn how to conduct a Shared Reading session as a reading companion is simply to jump in at the deep end and enjoy the unexpected effects you will undoubtedly experience!

Whoever wishes to know more about the finer points of being a reading companion can always seek guidance from Het Lezerscollectief. This organisation has wide ranging experience of the use of the Shared Reading methodology within the care context and understands the specific needs and questions of reading companions in the care sector.

The examples and testimonies in this book are all drawn from the experiences of trained Lezerscollectief reading companions. Together, they form a tight-knit learning network, whose members continue to meet regularly, even after they have completed their basic training, so that they can further refine their individual approaches and themselves benefit from the salutary effect of Shared Reading; benefits that they are then better able to pass on to their own reading groups.

More information about the work and the training courses organised by Het Lezerscollectief can be found at the back of the book.

As an alternative, it is also possible to first experience the power of Shared Reading by arranging an informal reading session for your family or friends (or by having them read aloud for you!), following which you can discuss what has been read. This will allow you to practice in a safe environment, in which you can practice and learn without the fear of making mistakes. In this way, you will soon sense what a discussion of a text involves and what kind of effect it can have. What types of questions stimulate a good dialogue? What kinds of things do you, as a listener, like to experience? Which kinds of approach do you find uncomfortable or even unpleasant? Having these personal experiences in the back of your mind serves as an ideal platform for later Shared Reading with your patients or clients.

Of course, there are one or two other crucial starting points for anyone who wants to become a good reading companion: a good store of empathy, love for literature, and the openness to allow yourself and your listeners to be surprised by the richness and the healing power for growth that sits hidden in stories and poems. Does this sound like you? Then what are we waiting for! Let's go!

1
Starting

On Liberty and Slavery

Alas! and am I born for this,
To wear this slavish chain?
Deprived of all created bliss,
Through hardship, toil and pain!

How long have I in bondage lain,
And languished to be free!
Alas! and must I still complain—
Deprived of liberty.

Oh, Heaven! and is there no relief
This side the silent grave—
To soothe the pain—to quell the grief
And anguish of a slave?

Come Liberty, thou cheerful sound,
Roll through my ravished ears!
Come, let my grief in joys be drowned,
And drive away my fears.

Say unto foul oppression, Cease:
Ye tyrants rage no more,
And let the joyful trump of peace,
Now bid the vassal soar.

Soar on the pinions of that dove
Which long has cooed for thee,
And breathed her notes from Afric's grove,
The sound of Liberty.

Oh, Liberty! thou golden prize,
So often sought by blood—
We crave thy sacred sun to rise,
The gift of nature's God!

Bid Slavery hide her haggard face,
And barbarism fly:
I scorn to see the sad disgrace
In which enslaved I lie.

Dear Liberty! upon thy breast,
I languish to respire;
And like the Swan unto her nest,
I'd like to thy smiles retire.

Oh, blest asylum—heavenly balm!
Unto thy boughs I flee—
And in thy shades the storm shall calm,
With songs of Liberty!

George Moses Horton

Breaking through patterns of habit

For people in need of care of one kind or another, starting with Shared Reading is by no means self-evident. Finding the energy that is necessary is not easy for people who often feel vulnerable and sluggish. Starting something new is like the first freshness of spring, when nature bursts back into life in all its glory and with full force. A season of possibilities and promise.

Moving into action, taking the initiative, getting something on the rails: if our life is going well, we can take things in our stride, confident that our momentum will carry us through. We can see where we want to go and set off resolutely along the path that will lead to the realisation of our dreams.

But this is not so easy for people who are sick or in need of care, whether in an institution or at home. They are often weighed down by baggage from the past and, to a greater or lesser extent, have reached the point of stagnation. Their life, either in whole or in part, seems to have come to a standstill or is at least slowing down. Simply through the necessity of being physically present in an institution for the purposes of care, whether resident or outpatient, the world of the patient or client is made smaller. Anyone who has to visit hospital three times a week for kidney dialysis is hardly in a position to make long-distance journeys…

To make matters worse, the structures in the care sector make it even more difficult to launch new initiatives. The need for economy has strangled creative thinking on more than one occasion. Moreover, care institutions like to stick to the routines and procedures that have proven their effectiveness over the years, sometimes at the expense of the specific needs of the individual patient. This means that patients find it increasingly hard to take the independent actions best suited to their condition. An older person in a care home or someone with a limitation who visits a day-care centre will find their hands tied by a fixed routine. Similarly, a patient in a psychiatric hospital or an adolescent in a youth rehabilitation facility will have a fairly inflexible weekly programme forced upon them. True, these routines and programmes contain a degree of variation – Tuesday morning: therapy, Wednesday afternoon: sport, Thursday morning: creativity, etc. – but in general terms it is probably fair to say that the activities offered to people in residential or semi-residential care of whatever kind cannot really be described as being full of adventure and exciting new discoveries.

Likewise, people who spend long periods at home because they are sick or recovering from burnout run the risk of stagnation and isolation. Even the mere prospect of having to engage in a new initiative is often enough to frighten them off. And the longer they stay at home, the harder it becomes to take the first step towards any new form of activity or change in the future. After months of illness or burnout, it takes courage to find your way back to the office or workfloor, not to mention a great deal of imaginative power to develop improved ways of working or to establish better interaction with your colleagues or boss. And what if you don't have the necessary courage and imagination? The care system will ensure that this person stays at home for an even longer period, because they are not yet 'ready' to return. And so they are pushed deeper and deeper into a vicious circle that becomes ever harder to break.

Shared Reading forces people to break out of their routine and to leave behind their standard patterns of behaviour. For an hour or perhaps a bit longer, it transports them to a world full of imagination and unforeseen opportunities. A powerful literary text contains various layers of possible meaning. A short story or poem is not a factual statement, but a magical box of tricks, overflowing with unexpected contents and dreams. A well-written text sparks off the imagination of its readers and listeners, and opens in their mind a large space that has many entrances and exits.

It is above all during the discussion of the texts that this new space becomes filled with new perspectives that suddenly become visible. Moreover, the same personage or the same event in a story is capable of numerous different interpretations. For some readers, this is a surprising discovery.

> In a temporary reading group, the short story *Two words* by Isabel Allende is read. The main character in the story is Belisa Crepusculario, a young woman who discovers the power of words and turns it into her profession. During a pause in the reading, the listeners exchange ideas about what kind of person Belisa really is.
>
> 'In my opinion, she is just full of hot air,' says Francine. Her tone is laconic, suggesting a degree of contempt for Belisa, as if she has just exposed her as being a fraud.
>
> A silence falls over the group. At the other side of the circle, someone offers a different view. 'But she is certainly enterprising,' suggests Hendrik. 'Surely that is something we can regard as a positive quality? She has made something of her life. She has been through so much, but has always managed to come out on top.' Others in the group agree. 'She makes use of what she finds on her way. That's smart. And it takes guts.' But Francine also has her supporters, who see Belisa as an odd kind of woman who is constantly pulling the wool over people's eyes.
>
> The conversation moves backwards and forwards in this manner for several minutes, until the reading companion decides the time has come to pick up the thread of the story.

When people are trapped in a fixed pattern of thought and can only see one route through life, engaging in a conversation about a literary text can often help them to see that there are alternative pathways. If I am afraid to return to work after a burnout, because I am terrified at the thought of a new confrontation with my boss, reading a story can perhaps help me to see that there are different ways in which you can assess and approach a person.

Wait a minute… If I can see Belisa not only as a charlatan, but also as an enterprising young woman, perhaps there is also another way I can look at my boss? The seed of a new idea has been planted, from which can grow a new plan of action. *Perhaps I can discuss things with my boss more, maybe even negotiate. Or just be friendlier towards him. Or maybe ask for a different work post in a quieter location…*

New and unexpected options reveal themselves, even if in the first instance these are no more than tentative possibilities. You consider them for a moment and then file them away in your memory, for a more detailed examination later on. Because change is something that takes time. Often, you only get there by taking a series of small steps over a longer period. And in most cases, it is the very first step that is the most difficult of all; after that, things tend to go more smoothly.

Inspired to take action

'A book is a dream that you hold in your hands.'

Neil Gaiman

Providing people with good quality care includes the obligation to offer them the space and the inspiration that will allow them to see new possibilities. You must also help them to find the courage that will allow them to explore and exploit those possibilities. People who are sick or hampered by a limitation need to reinvent themselves before they can move forward again in life.

An inspirational carer can give them a helpful push in the back that will persuade them to take that all-important first step on what might be a very long journey towards successful change. Moreover, the slowness of a person's recovery and healing may also mean that this journey is not always in keeping with society's expectations. Because society likes people who get on with things. Quick starters – people who dare and do – are generally admired. True, there are always some who jealously jeer at them from the sidelines, motivated by their own inability to be as decisive in their actions. But, as a rule, we praise those who are fast and confident, while we have little sympathy for those who fail to start at all or who for one reason or another find themselves at an impasse, so that they can move neither backwards or forwards. Of course, in theory there is a social safety net for these people who fail to find their way in the world, but there are always some who slip through the holes in this net. Men and women who suddenly find themselves isolated in the margins of society are quickly branded as failures, with only themselves to blame for their misfortune.

That being said, even people who are seemingly successful can suddenly find themselves paralysed by the pressure to continually perform; by high levels of expectation (their own or others'); by the conflict between what the person deep down truly wants and what he thinks is good, honourable and acceptable; or by concern about whether these parameters match his own image of himself and his social status.

Moreover, people who, because of illness or a mental or physical impediment, suddenly find themselves beyond the limits of normal social circulation are often confronted with the additional barriers created by their condition and its treatment or therapy. Dealing with this situation often demands so much energy that they can no longer see how they can initiate new action that will allow them to escape from their predicament. It is simply beyond them.

Following new pathways does indeed demand plenty of energy, courage and vision. If you want to see new opportunities, you need an open and receptive mind, allied to the imagination, to envisage new and creative solutions. Daring to follow 'the path less travelled' always involves the risk that you might get lost, but that is a risk you sometimes need to take. Because it also opens up the possibility that you will discover new horizons.

Shared Reading can help to inspire people to take action. Often, it can do this in a much freer way than classic care or therapy, because a reading session offers more open space, in which there is no pressure to perform and no expectation to make progress. You are just who you are. Present, listening, reading. Within this unforced atmosphere of freedom, texts can have the ability to inspire new ideas and dreams. Sometimes this inspiration might be found in small things, like a true-to-life description of nature that prompts a person to finally go for a walk in the woods again, after many months of isolation. But a text can also inspire people to make major, life-changing choices.

Marc has worked in education for twelve years. But he is finding it hard. Very hard. He always gets the most difficult classes with the most difficult pupils. As a result, he always needs to be on the lookout for their latest acts of mischief and he gets no support from his colleagues and his director, who all prefer to look the other way. Because of the pressure, Marc has been absent from school on a number of occasions, for increasingly longer periods. 'Just to get my breath back,' he calls it. But he is finding it harder and harder to motivate himself to continue his 'battle' against the rebels in his class. In fact, he no longer feels like a real teacher; more like a policeman. To help distract his mind and forget about his worries, Marc decides to join a reading group. He enjoys the relaxed atmosphere and the discussion of the texts with the other participants. Then one night, unexpectedly, a poem triggers something inside of him. The poem is *Sasja* by Ed Franck and it activates a thought that has been brewing at the back of his mind for quite some time: *'Wouldn't it be better for me if I simply changed jobs? Stop teaching at school and start up something on my own?'* Some weeks pass as Marc considers the answers to these questions, but he finally decides to take the plunge. He quits school and sets up his own business as a self-employed contractor. In the months and weeks that follow, Marc is transformed. His depression vanishes, to be replaced by a new optimism and enjoyment of life. His new work is challenging, but always interesting. In fact, business is so good that he now has employees of his own and together they form a strong and close-knit team. But Marc has never forgotten

> the poem that prompted the click in his mind. When he got home from the reading group that night, he stuck it on the mirror in his bedroom. And there it still hangs.

> I suggest that the only books
> That influence us are those for
> Which we are ready, and which
> Have gone a little further down
> Our particular path than
> We have yet gone ourselves
>
> *E.M. Forster in* Two Cheers for Democracy

Taking risks always involves a degree of adventure. Some people accept risks gladly and with verve; others run a million miles whenever they see a risk coming. The first group is typified by the many young start-ups we see in the economy today, companies that are bursting with creativity and a spirit of entrepreneurship. But start-ups that keep launching one new initiative after another threaten to be swamped by an unbridled growth, simply because they fail to take the necessary time for reflection.

Similarly, people can also sow the seeds of their own destruction if they continue to plough forward in an irresponsible and blinkered fashion, almost regardless of everyone and everything. Without pausing to see where we are and to look where we are going, we risk losing our way and draining all the energy from our batteries. But the opposite approach is equally unsatisfactory. Failing to dream and failing to act results in a passivity that actually rusts your batteries before you ever get a chance to use them.

Shared Reading can help people to find the right balance between burning out and spluttering to a standstill. Literary texts can help people to discover the surprising joy of the thoughts locked away inside their minds, whether they are readers or listeners. They stimulate the imagination and provide the inspiration for new ideas and new dreams. And dreams are the main drivers of action. A dream that is developed eventually becomes a plan.

But before this can happen, you first need to have the courage to confront and accept your immediate reality. This is not always possible for every patient or recipient of care. Sometimes their pain, physical or psychological, is so great that it demands all their attention. Even so, people suffering with chronic pain have told me that during a session of Shared Reading they temporarily forget their pain, or at least manage to push it into the background of their consciousness. Why? Because at last they have something else, something worthwhile, on which to focus: the story or poem that they read and the subsequent discussions about it with their fellow readers.

Literature opens the door on a world that has often been made narrow by pain and other limitations. It helps to create extra space, which makes it possible to explore other pathways that offer more than just the cares and worries of our normal daily routine. New variations on old patterns, unexpected perceptions, emotions that you have never previously experienced or allowed: access to all these things and so much more can be found through the simple reading and discussion of a piece of prose or poetry.

In the space created by a literary text, the reader feels like an explorer, moving beyond the boundaries of his or her known world. There, on the far side of the horizon of the everyday, awaits a land of dreams and imagination, just waiting to be discovered.

Dealing safely with the unpredictable

The trigger that prompts a person to take action can be found anywhere in and around a text. It might be a word that sparks off a memory or a finely phrased sentence that unlocks a particular aesthetic response, but it can just as easily be a difference of opinion with another reader about the text or the confirmation of your own thoughts by another reader who shares them.

Because we are all different, it is difficult to predict what kinds of text will unlock the hidden doors in people's minds. Words that can generate a powerful emotional reaction in one reader will have no effect on another reader, who may even find those same words to be trivial and banal. For this reason, it is not a good idea for reading companions to choose their texts with the specific intention of provoking this or that kind of reaction or effect. A series of success stories about dynamic winners to help people overcome their depression? Don't do it! On the contrary, a story about someone weighed down with a sense of failure or powerlessness can sometimes have a greater effect on a patient who is incapable of action, simply because of the greater feeling of recognition. But even that is by no means certain. There are no easy recipes for 'success'. It is much better simply to give the imagination of your readers free rein. Choose your text without preconceptions and just see how they react, in all their openness and unpredictability. That being said, an ideal sequence of texts over a number of different reading sessions should take account of the readers – what are their problems, what are their interests, what is their level of ability, etc. – but without ever trying to ram a particular 'salutary' message down their throats. The breakthrough is often to be found in an insignificant corner of a text, but it is impossible to predict which words will spark a reaction in which reader.

We all read and listen through our own particular filter. We see in a story or poem parallels with the things we are experiencing in our own lives. At the same time, this filter also serves as a blocker, hiding the things that we dislike in ourselves, the things that we do not want to talk about or let others see. Fortunately, however, it is precisely these inner demons that are given more space to manifest within the context of a reading group.

Moreover, we do not even need to make these demons explicitly clear to our fellow readers. Often it is enough just to sit and listen to the opinions of others and then compare them in silence with your own. If, for example, I realise that some people regard a personage in a story as being 'cute', while I am seething with fury at what I see as their deceit and hypocrisy, perhaps this will help me in my own mind to be a little more forgiving about the 'secret' aspects of my own personality that I regard with distaste.

A reading group offers a space for this kind of self-analysis that is different from therapy. In group therapy, the participants are expected to give direct comments on each other's thoughts and feelings. This kind of immediate response can often be experienced as harsh or even threatening by the person at whom it is directed. Individual therapy sessions can also have the same effect, with the full focus being placed on the client and his or her condition. Once again, the client is expected to respond; there is no opportunity to just sit quietly in a corner and think about the things that you would perhaps prefer not to put into words.

In Shared Reading sessions, people are free to take part in the discussion of the texts, but are not obliged to do so. This offers the more reticent readers a feeling of safety. When someone is unexpectedly triggered by a particular sequence of words, but does not immediately know how to deal with the resulting emotions, a reading group allows them to withdraw briefly into themselves, so that they can let what has just happened sink in. And even when people do want to talk and discuss, what they express is their reactions to the text, not their reactions to each other as individuals.

True, this can sometimes result in people putting forward and exchanging their personal opinions, opinions that can often clash. But in the final analysis the text is always there as a kind of safe landing ground: when the discussion risks getting out of hand, the reading companion can always gently reassert control over the situation by referring back to where the discussion first began: the text.

Tips for practice

'No, no, the adventures first. Explanations take such a dreadful time.'

Lewis Carroll, The Adventures of Alice

1. Make clear agreements with the reading companion and with your organisation and place of work about what is expected of whom. Who does what? Who reserves the reading room? Who arranges the chairs, makes copies of the texts, etc? Who informs the readers when and where the session will take place and who, if necessary, collects them?
2. Make the space where the reading session takes place as comfortable and as welcoming as possible. Do not use spaces that are otherwise used as therapy or treatment spaces. With a few chairs in a circle and a supply of tea, coffee and biscuits on a table it is possible to create an atmosphere that is warm and homely, in which the readers can feel relaxed.
3. Always give the participants a copy of the text that is to be read.
4. Start and finish the reading session at the agreed times. Respect that period that the readers have made free to take part in the Shared Reading process.

2
Growing

Invictus

Out of the night that covers me,
   Black as the Pit from pole to pole,
I thank whatever gods may be
   For my unconquerable soul.
In the fell clutch of circumstance
   I have not winced nor cried aloud.
Under the bludgeonings of chance
   My head is bloody, but unbowed.
Beyond this place of wrath and tears
   Looms but the Horror of the shade,
And yet the menace of the years
   Finds, and shall find, me unafraid.
It matters not how strait the gate,
   How charged with punishments the scroll,
I am the master of my fate:
   I am the captain of my soul.

William Ernest Henley

Growing: a multi-dimensional process

In a care environment, growth is often in the first instance a matter of recovery: the healing not only of physical wounds, but also mental and emotional scars. People who are dependent on care for a long time often reduce their own expectations about what is possible in terms of their progress or healing. Recovery can be slow, and those suffering from a chronic illness or faced by a permanent limitation sometimes abandon hope of any fundamental improvement. Perhaps this is because society as a whole has a tendency to evaluate progress in external terms. How much more can person X do this week in comparison with last week? How much headway has been made and how many more sessions will be needed before the patient can be discharged or the therapy ended?

This is approach is too simple: growth has many different nuances. For example, growth can occur if people ask themselves deeper questions and become more sensitive as a result. But you cannot show this kind of growth on a curve. It finds its expression in subtle ways in a person's daily life. In the way patients deal with an off-day or make new plans for the near (or even slightly more distant) future. In the way they interact with other people – fellow-patients, carers, passers-by and chance encounters. In the way they look at themselves and are able, for instance, to display leniency and patience in their pursuit of their personal evolution. This is not a predictable linear process.

Inner growth is always erratic. It does not move forwards in a straight line. We can measure the physical growth of children by marking a succession of lines on a wall, so that we can see in black and white how they are gradually getting bigger and bigger. But inner growth as a person cannot be measured in that straightforward way. It not only moves upwards, but also inwards and outwards. It not only has height, but also depth. You can compare it to a tree. A tree sinks its roots deep into the ground, whilst at the same time spreading its branches higher and higher, adding a new ring to its girth with each passing year. And it is the same with people: they grow in different dimensions simultaneously. The force that drives this growth is the life-giving warmth of summer. The warmth of the sun, transformed into warmth in the heart of a human being. Love, bonding with others, passion, empathy… It is heart energy that makes us the social creatures we are. Delight and unrestrained enjoyment are an essential part of growth. It is this same strength of heart that gives us the courage to show ourselves to the outside world: we express ourselves; we reveal ourselves in all our facets; we jump on the world's stage and shout: 'Here I am!'

Or that, at least, is how growth should take place in ideal circumstances, free and unhindered. Unfortunately, real life does not always run so smoothly. There are ups and downs. Somewhere along our path we will face setbacks, so that we no longer dare to reveal ourselves openly or to connect with others.

Some people are able to contextualise these setbacks, seeing them as part of the beauty of life. Others find it more difficult to come to terms with the damage such setbacks often cause. Of course, it is true that some people's setbacks are more dramatic and have more far-reaching consequences than others. It is equally true that people have differing abilities to cope with misfortune. The result is a varied human landscape, in which some people thrive and are visible from afar, while others, wounded and afraid, retreat into a corner where they hope that life will be less harsh. In this latter group, personal growth is almost non-existent.

There is no point in attempting to force people to grow or to jettison the difficult baggage they are carrying from the past. You cannot direct or control growth. What you can do, however, is to create favourable conditions in which growth can occur; conditions in which people will feel comfortable and where they will be able to develop more of their potentiality.

It is also important to pay attention to these matters in a care setting. In some areas this already happens. People with a physical or mental limitation are stimulated to develop within the space created by their own abilities and possibilities. In long-stay psychiatric departments, for example, efforts are made to develop stronger social and emotional skills. In other words, personal growth and development are clear objectives of the hospitalisation process.

In other fields, however, much less space for growth is offered. This is often the case, for example, in residential care homes. The higher level of physical care that older people need frequently results in a corresponding lack of attention for emotional and mental stimulation. Financial constraints and time pressure are key factors in creating this unsatisfactory situation. The available people and resources are committed first and foremost to providing basic care.

In these circumstances, Shared Reading with patients or clients, organised and assisted either by a member of staff or by an external volunteer, opens up a range of interesting possibilities. A reading group offers people low-threshold opportunities for growth within a pleasing framework that is divorced from high-cost and high-intensity therapeutic interventions.

Shared Reading as a free space for growth

Shared Reading creates a free space in which growth can occur. Not 'must' occur, but 'can' occur. There is no expectation of progress. However, it is precisely this freedom and lack of expectation that often unlocks something in people, so that unexpected and extraordinary things can result.

The informal and unforced nature of a literary text is a basic condition for growth. The thoughts of the reader and the listener are free to roam in whatever direction they please. During the discussion sessions in the breaks between the readings the participants do not need to worry about giving the 'right' answer. There is no right or wrong answer. There is only the reaction of the individual participants to the story or poem they have heard. And the resulting conversations can sometimes lead to remarkable outcomes.

Jan had been coming to the reading group with his wife Veerle for some time. Their house doctor had told them about Shared Reading. At their first session Veerle explained that Jan could no longer talk. 'He had a stroke and lost all power of speech. So he won't be able to say anything. Not because he doesn't want to, but because he can't.'

It sounded like a court verdict, but the group came to know Jan as someone who was silently present and nodded politely in response to the words of others.

One evening, the group read the story *Duiverke* (The Pigeon) by Geertrui Daem. The person in charge of the session was sitting next to Jan. He soon became aware that Jan was powerfully affected by the text. The world of pigeon racing and the personage of Ronny Waeymeersch in particular seemed to unlock something inside of him.

During the second break in the reading, Jan became more and more agitated and suddenly emitted two complete sentences, two complete rows of words, one after the other. It was his reaction to the events in the story, based on his own personal sense of engagement to what he had heard. What's more, he spoke with a total naturalness of expression, as though he had never been robbed of his ability to speak.

How does it happen that people can achieve a breakthrough or a burst of growth in their inner development? And what role can Shared Reading play in this process? What are the key factors in its ability to unlock seemingly closed doors? Is it the comfortable atmosphere of the reading space, so that the participants no longer regard themselves as patients or clients and are freed from the burden of their medical condition? Is it the calming voice of the reader, which relaxes the listeners and reminds them of the enjoyment of being read to as a child? These elements are certainly beneficial for encouraging growth. When you are in a relaxed frame of mind, you are much more capable of growing than when you are under stress. Stress means that you are unconsciously in a non-stop 'flight-or-fight' mode, so that nothing new can reach you.

But there is more to it than that. If we dig deeper, it becomes clear that the most important aspect of Shared Reading is its ability to increase a person's inner space. This is the space that someone has available for their own thoughts and feelings; in other words (to use the jargon), their mental-emotional space. Shared Reading stimulates the expansion of this space in two different ways. Firstly, it makes use of a literary text, which creates a zone of experience in which the participants are confronted with new thoughts and sensations. Secondly, the breaks in the reading sessions provide a setting in which the experience of those thoughts and sensations can be discussed. Together, these two elements have the potential to create magic.

The story as a zone of experience

'Literature is only literature if its author also fails to fully understand the text.'

György Konrád

A good story creates a zone of experience. The story is developed in a linear manner, because the writer needs to get his story told coherently, but in the zone generated by and around the story everything happens at the same time. You sense instinctively when a story is a good story or a strong story, a story that has different layers of meaning. It is impossible to summarise it in a few sentences, because you cannot compress and explain its many different nuances and subtleties.

A good story embodies the genius of the author. It contains so much narrative power that it unfolds and occupies a space in your head, even if it deals with subject matter to which you are unable to relate directly in your daily life, such as magical events or science fiction.

People who regularly take part in Shared Reading often say that they feel as though a new world has been opened up for them. A three-dimensional world in which they can explore and have new experiences, running parallel with the events being described by the author. Within the zone of experience created by the story, each reader and listener develops their own alternative story line, coloured by their own personal emotions and thoughts in response to what is happening in the text.

Good stories enlarge your own inner space, so that you come into contact with themes that are unfamiliar to you and with which you have no direct experience. A writer who is able to paint a vivid word picture of 'war' can give you the feeling that you are actually experiencing what it is like to be involved in such a war. Stories can take you to another time, place and culture, immersing you in them completely. In this way, stories do indeed open up a new world.

The space created by the story increases in relation to the intensity of emotion with which the reader is able to navigate through that space. A good writer does everything possible to expand the boundaries of the mental-emotional space in which the story takes place. The layered nature of the text can lead to moments of amazement or even synchronicity, which suddenly allow the reader to see parallels with his own life.

At such moments it almost seems as if time stands still. You sense something timeless entering into your personal experience. It is the feeling you get when you look at a star-studded sky on a clear night or during a relaxing evening in good company, when you suddenly think: 'This is perfect'. It only lasts for a few seconds, and then it is gone.

This kind of experience can also be generated by reading literature. You cannot predict such experiences in advance; they occur spontaneously at moments when you engage with the deeper layers of the text and take them into yourself. This dramatically increases your inner space, as a result of which your thoughts and emotions become clearer, simply because they have more room in which to develop and unfold.

In many cases, the writer will not have consciously foreseen this effect. Powerful literary texts contain layers of meaning that go beyond rational appreciation. We understand these layers intuitively and are able to link their more profound aspects to elements in our own lives. These are rare and precious moments, which allow us to grow and deepen our awareness, simply by reading or listening to a piece of literature.

The conversation space during the breaks in the reading

'Reading is thinking with someone else's head.'

Arthur Schopenhauer

During the breaks in the reading of the text, the reading companion asks a number of open questions about its content, with the aim of starting off a conversation. The participants are not obliged to take part in this conversation. If they want to join in, they can. If they want to just listen, that is fine, too.

Even so, these breaks always bring the participants into contact and connection with each other. They exchange experiences, ideas and opinions about the text and in this way learn from each other, even if they do not take an active part in the discussion.

At first glance, such discussions may seem like nothing special to an outsider, but what happens to the participants is truly remarkable and makes possible their further inner growth. To explain this more fully, we need to take a closer look at a phenomenon that exists inside the human brain: its network of mirror neurons.

Mirror neurons

Mirror neurons are a set of special neurons – nerve cells in the brain – that help us to learn new behaviour through imitation. Research into mirror neurons is relatively recent. By monitoring the activity of the brain, using amongst other things EEG and fMRI (functional Magnetic Resonance Imaging), researchers can see what happens inside our head when we interact with others. This in turn sheds light on what happens when the participants in Shared Reading talk to each other and explains how they are able to learn from each other.

Neurons are connected to each other in networks. Mirror neurons are activated (i.e., they fire off electric impulses to the next cell in the network) whenever we do something or have the intention to do that something or see someone else doing it. If I want to pick up a pen from the table, my mirror neurons are activated from the moment I formulate that intention. In my head, I have already made the necessary movement before I do it physically. When I see someone else reach for the pen, the same process occurs: the neurons that are necessary to perform the movement are likewise activated. In my mind, I imitate the action being performed by the other person.

The origin of this mechanism is to be found in our evolutionary biology. The more involved or interested you are in something, the more effectively the mirror neurons in your brain will be activated. When an ape sees another ape in the same group peel a nut, the same zones in the brain of the watching ape are activated as in the brain of the ape doing the peeling. If the action you are watching is an action in which you are less closely involved or interested, your mirror neurons will be correspondingly less active.

Mirror neurons are not only activated for **motor functions**, but also for **emotions**. If I see someone register disgust because of an unpleasant smelling fruit, I will start to feel the same disgust as well. This reflex will be even stronger if that someone is someone I know well or is a member of my group.

This is a remnant of our evolution as a species. Copying what you see happening to others was part of our human survival strategy. If I see that a member of our group has become ill through eating a particular kind of berry, I know that I need to avoid those berries in future. If an unknown person makes a sudden hand movement in my direction, I need to be able to assess immediately whether or not this is a friendly gesture or the prelude to an attack.

As a result of this mirror activity in our brain, we can feel the emotions that others feel, simply by observing them. Of course, this process is more effective if there is something more overtly physical to observe. If you are looking at someone who feels disgust, it is easier to feel the same if he screws up his face with distaste rather than if he simply shakes his head. Nevertheless, the brain is capable of registering even the smallest physiological changes in others, so that a similar emotional response can be activated, albeit at a lower intensity.

Our mirroring also begins when we see **physical pain**. If we see someone put his hand too close to a flame, we instinctively pull back our own hand. Similarly, our mirror neurons are also triggered in response to **moral codes**. When someone offends my moral code – for example, by failing to keep a promise – I find that difficult to accept. When I see someone offend my moral code in respect of someone else – for example, if I see my neighbour cheating on his wife – I find this equally difficult to accept.

Our mirror neurons not only mirror behaviour and emotions, but also the things we **remember** or **imagine**. If I am recalling the memories of my last winter holiday, in my mind I suddenly find myself once again skiing down the snow-covered slopes. And the same is true for sportsmen and women preparing for competition: by imagining the race they need to run and the movements they need to make in very concrete terms, they activate the mirror neurons in their brain in precisely the same manner as they would when actually performing those movements.

But it goes even further than that – and this is where the link with literature comes in. We also mirror **images**, **imaginary constructions**, **situations** and **contexts**. In other words: if we read a story or poem, our mirror neurons immediately spring into action. We empathise with what the fictive character in the story or poem experiences, just as we would with a real live person in the same situation. His fear, misery, hope and despair become our fear, misery, hope and despair. In our thoughts we can climb mountains with others, swim oceans and commit crimes with them. In particular with texts that aim specifically to engage our senses, it is easy to become totally involved in the story being told.

It is the same when our moral codes are broken in a story: our mirror neurons are activated to reflect our displeasure. If I am angry at a character in a story because he wants to find a lover for his wife, because he himself is hopelessly in love with a much younger woman, this indicates that his actions go beyond the boundaries of what is acceptable to my moral code.

You might even go so far as to say that the activities of our mirror neurons make it possible for us to 'read' each other. This perception does not always need to be visual: we can also react to what we perceive with our other senses – what we hear, taste, smell or feel. In this way, we can experience and sympathise with what we see happening to others. In short: we develop **empathy**. We can vividly imagine what the other person must be feeling, because we repeat the same actions and sensations in our head, and all simply by looking at the person in question.

This process allows us to better understand each other. Because I can see someone else's sorrow, I can sympathise with that person and acknowledge the sorrow he feels. And because this allows us to better understand each other, we can move on to relationships of a higher order. This is how we develop our social intelligence and how we learn to care for each other.

The mirror neuron system is closely connected with our sympathetic or autonomous nervous system and it **remains active throughout our life**. As a result, we can learn from each other until the day we die!

So what exactly do mirror neurons have to do with Shared Reading? A great deal. During the processes of reading and listening and in particular during the exchange sessions in the reading breaks, our mirror neurons are hard at work. On the one hand, they allow us to reflect on the content of the text: identifying with the characters, feeling approval or disapproval for their actions, sympathising with their dilemmas, sharing their emotions, etc. On the other hand, we can also reflect on the opinions of others about the text, as expressed during the midbreak discussions. And these opinions can differ significantly. What is 'not done' for one person might be regarded as acceptable or even admirable by someone else. While for me the story of *Judith* by Charles Ducal about the love of a married father for a younger woman clearly crossed a moral boundary, I had much less of a problem with the story *Powdered Snow* by Tobias Wolff, in which a man made a mockery of legal authority. In this latter story, the man in question cleverly lured away the police manning a roadblock on a snow-covered road, so that he could continue his journey. Many of my fellow readers found this behaviour outrageous – 'You just don't do that kind of thing!' – whereas I thought the man's actions were smart and amusing.

During the discussion of literary texts people come face to face with their true selves. By interacting with others, they discover the boundaries of their own inner world. And slowly, little by little, these boundaries are opened up and extended: in part by the author, who transports them to the world of the story or poem; in part by their fellow readers, who sometimes have very different opinions from their own about what is right, wrong, funny, disgusting, over the top, inspirational, etc. By reflecting on the text and on each other, people experience a wide range of different emotions and allow themselves to examine modes of thought that they might never have allowed otherwise. Someone who has been at daggers drawn with a parent or ex-partner for years might for the first time in his life be confronted with the idea of possible forgiveness. Simply by reading about a character in a story who has shown such forgiveness, the door to a new scenario is opened up in the imagination of the reader. New paths of action and ways of thought are revealed. Whether or not the person concerned will follow one of these paths – in this case, for example, by renewing contact with his parent or ex-partner – is another matter. But at least the possibility now exists, and all because he has shared the road that leads to forgiveness with a fictive character in a story.

As a further 'bonus', by reflecting on the reactions of our fellow readers we also develop a better understanding and greater empathy for each other. I might be appalled by the idea of a man who looks for a new partner for his wife, even if only in thought, whereas the person sitting next to me might see this as a sign of compassion, since the man, even in his infidelity, is still concerned for his wife and does not wish for her to be left behind alone. This compassionate interpretation of the story sets me thinking and persuades me to consider a different perspective. At that moment, I am mirroring the compassion displayed by my fellow reader and can gradually begin to see his point. Just briefly, I can stand with my thoughts in the place where that compassion exists, even though I might not agree with it. But at least I am testing it out. And by experiencing this alternative perspective, I slowly come to see my fellow reader in a new light, simply as someone who has different views to my own, and no longer as an 'opponent' who I must 'convert' to my own way of thinking. In short, I have become more understanding and less judgemental.

Interactions of this kind during Shared Reading can have a powerful healing effect. Not only for the individual participants in the reading group, whose mental and emotional worlds are significantly expanded, but also for the relationships between those participants. Via the reading of literary texts, people learn how to take in and digest different perspectives that might not be their own, rather than simply dismissing these perspectives as nonsense. This leads to a growth in empathy and mutual understanding. Just as importantly, it also leads to greater self-understanding, since it allows people to reassess and correct their existing ways of thinking. Ideas that were once black-and-white are now invested with a new degree of nuance, so that other possible interpretations of the same facts, events and personages are now considered. This expansion of their thinking and feeling is highly beneficial.

'My girls group was not exactly good when it came to empathy. Sometimes it really got me down. I put in so much effort and all I got in return was cold indifference. Suddenly one day, there was a breakthrough.

I read *The Boy Who Ate an Oakwood Chair* by the Dutch author Edward Van de Vendel. At a break in the reading one of the girls said, referring to the text: "That's impossible, dying with a smile on your lips." Recently, my mother had passed away and our parting was serene and peaceful. As a result, I told the group that such a thing was indeed possible. That when someone has finished with life and is able to leave it behind, with the feeling of having lived it to the full, a final last smile is by no means out of the question.

The group reacted emotionally. Not only the girl who had made the comment, but all the others as well. Within seconds, everyone had tears in their eyes. Did this turn the tide? And was this sharing of emotions necessary to achieve it?

Perhaps. In any event, the last few sessions were fantastic, with lots of outspoken opinions and serious discussions, but wholly devoid of their previous coolness. As they were leaving after the final session, they all asked: "Are there new sessions next year…?" That's girls for you!'

Ina, reading companion

Expanding the mental-emotional space

In the space created by the story or poem, we undergo new experiences in a world that the author has called into being with words, often in a highly layered manner. By empathising with and experiencing other people's perspectives in discussions about the text, our sympathy for and understanding of those others increases, whilst also softening the way we look at ourselves. The combination of these two processes significantly expands mental-emotional space. We have more room for new thoughts and feelings, which we have never previously allowed or tested.

This mental expansion is good. All of us – young or old, healthy or infirm – are urgently in need of a greater emotional space. Society does not currently provide us (at least not sufficiently) with the means by which we can create this additional space for ourselves. Today, we live in a world that is primarily two-dimensional. We spend large parts of every day looking at computers, tablets, television and other forms of image projection. These images suggest depth, but this is not the same as actually experiencing it. In this two-dimensional world, many of our interactions with others have been drastically simplified. Many people now have hundreds of Facebook friends, but hardly know anyone in real life.

In our superficial society there is a real and growing need for increased space in which to express our thoughts and emotions, so that we can reflect, fantasise, be creative, and develop new and authentic connections with others.

This need is perhaps greatest in people who are receiving care. They each live with a form of limitation; either a lack of proper development or a physical, emotional or psychological deficiency. People feel this limitation most keenly in their mental-emotional space, often much more than in their physical space. The majority express this by saying that they *feel* limited.

> Michel lost his right foot and the lower part of his leg in an accident at work. Initially, he was devastated by the thought that he was maimed for the rest of his days. His head was constantly full of the most frightful words associated with his condition: 'handicapped', 'invalid', 'cripple', 'disabled', etc. His mood soon became sombre and his actions passive. He seldom went anywhere and found it impossible to pick up the threads of his old life.

> Until one day he met a friend at a Christmas market. It was bitterly cold and his friend was stamping his feet to keep warm. Almost without thinking, the friend said: 'You've only got half the problem with the cold that I have!' There was a tense moment of silence – following which they both burst out laughing. Michel suddenly realised that there were advantages to his situation. Over a few beers, he even went on to name more of them, spicing his comments with some of his old humour.
>
> That evening, a friend's simple comment helped him to escape from his limiting sense of self-pity. The next morning he phoned his boss to ask when he could start back at work.

In education, care & support, and therapy

Our present-day society is only partly able to meet our need for a greater mental-emotional space. The education and training that we give to our young people nowadays is to a large degree focused on increasing the extent of their **mental space**. Their intellects are nourished and shaped. However, education pays little attention to their emotional space.

Care and support functions in all their many different forms – parents who care for children, people who care for a sick member of their family – help to make good this deficiency by concentrating primarily on developing the **emotional space** of their charges. People in care situations can make mistakes and these mistakes are corrected, but without losing the love of the people who care for them. They are given room to deal with their emotions. They can be angry or sad and sometimes lose control over their emotions completely: everything is accepted and tolerated in the same spirit of love and care.

However, what is often lacking is some form of dialogue to discuss and interpret those emotions. Helping care receivers to shape the mental framework for their emotions, so that they can give those emotions a proper place, is not generally a prominent part in these kinds of care relationships.

Therapy increases or repairs the **mental-emotional space** as part of a single process. Providing it is good therapy. Therapy presupposes a therapeutic contract between someone with a care need and someone who has the necessary competence to answer that need. The person with the care need is assumed to be prepared to give the therapist insight into his life, in order to establish the precise nature of the need. It is also assumed that the person in need will thereafter do what is necessary to achieve the desired therapeutic effect: by exploring the origins of the behavioural patterns relating to the problem; by examining the nature of all the influencing factors and by searching for new strategies to deal with problem situations; by practising calmer emotions and new modes of behaviour that will help to cope with similar situations, should they arise in the future.

This is a complex, lengthy and (consequently) expensive process. As a result, most therapies never get this far. In part, because most patients will not or cannot allow it. The large majority of people want to be relieved of their condition – whether physical or psychological – with the least effort and at the lowest cost. Acute physical problems can usually be treated quickly and without too much expense and bother. But all chronic conditions, both physical and psychological, result in long-term symptoms and therefore inevitably involve a wide range of associated thoughts and emotions. Each of these thoughts and emotions reduces the size of the mental-emotional space in which the client finds himself. They eat away at his self-image and hinder his former ability to think and feel freely. *'I will never get better... I will never be rid of this pain... This condition runs in my family... I need to be careful... I hope that it doesn't get worse...' People are often negatively affected more by their oppressive emotions and thoughts than by the actual nature of their condition.*

People often fail to realise that these thoughts and feelings about their condition not only diminish their physical space – the space in which they live – but also their mental space – the space in which they think. This persists until they rediscover the experience of space inside their head, like Michel in the example above. He rediscovered his sense of humour thanks to the friend's joke, as a result of which he was able to reoccupy his former mental space. In spite of his lasting physical limitation, mentally he now felt that he once again had both feet on the ground and was able to 're-start' his life the very next day.

Likewise, people often fail to realise that they do not have space within their thoughts and emotions for a particular theme. For example, a person who has a problem with authority and resists it with all his might has no place in his emotional space for a healthy relationship with authority figures. As soon as someone tries to exercise authority over him, he disconnects. Others might find it difficult to make space for a broken romance. Or for a physical limitation. Or for old age. These people have never reflected on these themes and refuse even to allow their possibility in their thoughts and emotions.

When a person's insight into his blind spot increases, because he is repeatedly confronted with it in different circumstances and therefore gradually becomes increasingly aware of his own role in its creation, his mental and emotional space in respect of the difficult theme expands significantly. In other words, this insight is beneficial.

Unfortunately, most people do not spontaneously engage in the kind of self-reflection that leads to insight. The circumstances that confront us with our blind spot are often very hard to deal with, because they relate so closely to our own behaviour. Every therapist will be familiar with the resistance to insightful dialogue shown by clients who wish to avoid the painful process of self-examination.

In Shared Reading

Like therapy, Shared Reading increases the mental-emotional space as part of a single process. However, it does so in a different manner. Because of the clever way in which the author develops the story line and because the text is read out slowly (reading aloud is six times slower than reading by sight), the story and its themes remain well fixed in the memory. In the breaks during the reading, these themes are discussed seriously and the participants exchange their thoughts, empathically and with respect for each other's point of view and experience of the text. This leads to the creation of new paths in their neurology, in their mental and emotional space, which also remain well fixed in their memory.

This effect is lasting. Because the participants' mirror neurons reflect on imaginary characters, this means that the participants need to actively imagine the story, building on the elements offered to them by the imagination of the author during the reading. For the human brain, this is a much more active process than undergoing therapy and it also results in a more intense learning process.

Moreover, a text also has more layers of meaning, which encourages more intense associative processes in the brain. As a result, the connection of themes in the story to themes in daily life usually occurs in a series of steps. The other participants generate a series of different associations, which all make possible further alternative connections with day-to-day life.

After the reading session, the participants take home copies of the texts that have been read, so that they can read them again. This strengthens new associations and insights even more. In contrast, the wise words of a therapist are often forgotten – or at least fade – as soon as the client walks out of the door. People often think back on the pleasant reading experiences they have had and can frequently recall the passages that made a particularly strong impression. They know exactly who said what and what response this evoked in them. Consequently, the expansion of their mental-emotional space does not end when the book is closed at the end of a reading session, but continues in the outside world.

> 'The reading from *The Art of War* by Sun Tzu occupied my thoughts for days. Especially the passage in which the general refused to allow the emperor to protect his courtesan after she had disobeyed him. The natural and forceful way in which the general punished her kept flitting through my mind. Severe, but oh so effective!
>
> In an instant, my responsibility became clear to me. I knew exactly how I would deal with my father's protégés in the company. Firmly and consistently.'
>
> *Kurt, second-generation company owner and participant in a group trajectory for burnout*

The therapeutic power of Shared Reading

Shared Reading has a therapeutic effect without the use of formal therapeutic techniques. Thanks to the power of imagination, freedom and creativity, the participants in reading sessions can grow in ways that are easier to achieve and often seem safer than classic therapy.

Imagination

The reading of texts aloud during Shared Reading sessions leaves plenty of room for the participants to exercise their own imagination. For preference, the reader should read in a neutral tone, which should be sufficiently vivid but without being overly emphatic, so that some of the spaces in the story still need to be filled in by those listening. Reading aloud is not the same as acting. Quite the contrary.

By leaving space for personal interpretation, the reader gives the listeners the opportunity to use their own creativity. If a mother gets angry in the text, the reader does not need to make her shout. Each participant paints his or her own picture. A participant who grew up in a family where shouting was the norm will immediately visualise a mother with a loud voice in his mind, whereas another participant whose mother expressed her anger in an icy stillness will mentally project this same childhood image.

In this respect, literature offers greater freedom than film or television, where the personages are clearly delineated by the director. When reading or listening to literature, people are to a much greater extent the directors of their own imagination. Because the mirror neurons in your brain reflect on what is happening in the text, you produce a whole range of mental images that match your own experience world. In this way, every participant in a Shared Reading session takes part in the story in his or her own way.

Of course, this creative contribution also occurs when a person reads in silence. But the most interesting aspect of Shared Reading is the fact that this process is linked to what is happening in the group (or reading duo). By exchanging impressions and experiences during the breaks in the reading, the participants discover how others have filled in the blanks in the story inside their own heads. In this way, it is possible that someone might realise for the very first time that there are more types of angry mothers than the one with which he is familiar from his own life. By placing people's different experiences alongside each other, it is possible to add nuance to images that might otherwise be traumatic or painful. As a result, the participants also learn that there are different ways of responding to trauma and sadness – whether it relates to angry mothers or to something else that cuts even more deeply into the soul.

Beyond the pain point

Is it not possible (I hear you ask) that the participants in a reading session end up traumatising each other through the sharing of their painful personal experiences? Might it not happen that someone who is already depressed as a result of a bad relationship with an angry mother is pushed even deeper into depression? Is it really responsible to discuss these things with people who are often vulnerable? Yes, it is.

The power of the discussion moments during the reading breaks is that the story subsequently continues. The participants do not explore these painful experiences for hours on end, but after a few minutes pick up the thread of the text. Put simply: they encounter a mother in the story, are given a brief opportunity to reflect on their relationship with their own mother… and then they move on. The trauma or pain spot is not the end point. Perhaps for the very first time, someone who has been deeply hurt as a result of a bad relationship with his mother will not remain locked in the painful grip of his emotions, but will take a new step forwards, so that he can see how the story will develop.

This is one of the beneficial effects of Shared Reading: the participants halt briefly at the place where their pain resides, but then leave it behind and continue their journey. This is the difference between a reading session and therapy. Most forms of therapy involve a detailed examination of the client's personal history, searching for the cause of his condition. The same ground is covered and reframed over and over again. Once it is understood how the condition has arisen, a carefully considered therapeutic plan is drawn up. This plan is highly targeted and structured, with step-by-step objectives, and takes the problem as its starting point. For many clients, this process is too slow and too intense.

The focus in the Shared Reading process is not fixed on personal conditions and disorders. It makes no difference whether a person taking part has chronic back pain or is suffering from loneliness. The story leads each participant into a virtual space: the space of his own imagination. Within this space everyone experiences his own personal interpretation of the story. If the story involves dealing with a painful event, each participant will feel his own pain, whether physical or emotional. Some of the participants may be willing to talk about this during one of the breaks, but at an appropriate moment the reading companion will refocus attention on the text.

Because the author continues to develop his story, a kind of evolution within the group occurs, generating a change in or a solution for the themes to which the participants can relate personally. The twists and turns in the story transport the listeners through the experience world created by the author, guiding them first towards and then beyond their own themes, always moving them forwards in a highly creative manner.

Flexible distance for difficult themes

During the reading breaks, the reading companion has an important role to play. He must decide when the discussion has lasted long enough, so that the moment has come to return to the text. This is something that requires careful thought and respect for the needs of the participants. Not everyone feels inclined to share their experiences and under no circumstances should people be invited or put under pressure to do so; not in a group and not as a one-to-one reading partner. Some people will wish to say nothing about their relationship with their mother, perhaps because their experience is too painful for words. Others will say nothing because their relationship with their mother is good, so that they feel they have nothing meaningful to contribute.

For this reason, the reading companion must avoid the temptation to go around each of the participants, asking them in turn to say something about their mother (or whatever else the theme might be). The focus must always remain on the text. This is the starting point and the finishing point for all discussions during the reading breaks.

This approach gives the participants a feeling of comfort and security. It allows them to decide for themselves how close to or how far from the theme under discussion they wish to get. As Professor Frank Hakemulder, researcher in media and cultural sciences at the University of Utrecht, has put it: 'As a reader, we weave our way into and out of the story. We are constantly travelling backwards and forwards between the fictional world and the real world.'

Just as someone who reads a book in private always has the option to close it if its contents become too upsetting, so each participant in a Shared Reading session is free to take a step back if the story being read comes too close to his own personal situation. Everyone is a liberty to identify with or to distance themselves from the characters in the reading. Yet even the people who take no active part in the mid-break discussions will no doubt have formed their own ideas about the theme in their thoughts and might even be conducting a virtual conversation in the safety of their own head. At the same time, these silent ones can also enjoy and learn from the conversations that the others in the group are having. For example, they may discover that another participant has managed to find the right words to describe their situation or to take steps forward in the inner process of healing, steps for which they, until now, had not been ready.

People who take part in Shared Reading appreciate this freedom and the fact that they can distance themselves in this way from their own problems. This was the conclusion of a survey conducted by The Reader organisation in 2017. The participants in a reading group were asked to comment on their experience of Shared Reading. Of the fourteen participants, six had had therapy or were still following it. All six said that they preferred the sessions with the reading group to their sessions with the psychiatrist. They thought that Shared Reading had more personal and emotional content than therapy and focused less on negative themes and problems. As a result, it did not give them the feeling that they were in the group because they were 'sick'. Instead, Shared Reading offered them a creative breathing space that had nothing to do with being a patient or client. They were simply present as readers with a complete history as a person and were free to decide what parts of that history they wished to share.

'There are millions of people in the world, but no one can know what another person is feeling inside. Everyone stands alone and must single-handedly navigate the storms of life. At Shared Reading, everyone has a chance to have their say after each chapter. It is interesting to hear and compare other opinions.

I can recognise myself in many of the stories, so that I no longer feel such a loner. I also get the chance to ventilate my feelings. I discover myself and others, gaining a new view of the world that makes me feel good. At moments like that I feel that I am making progress, because it is damned difficult to escape from the habits of a lifetime that have been forced upon us.'

Frans, a participant in a reading group for psychologically vulnerable people

Embracing the shadow side and unreachable experiences

'The wound is the place where the Light enters you.'

Rumi

A wide variety of themes are covered by Shared Reading. The participants meet regularly – weekly, fortnightly or at some other agreed frequency – and read different texts. A single session usually covers a short story and a poem, so that each session forms a coherent whole.

Each short story and poem highlights a different theme, which means that sooner or later every participant will be confronted with a theme in which he can recognise himself or with which he might even be struggling to cope. One week you read about someone who rashly falls head over heels in love, while the next week you read about the loss of a child. In other words, the readings chosen by the reading companion deal with life in all its aspects.

Every participant experiences the texts in a different manner, coloured by the way he approaches life in general and by what has happened to him, both good and bad, in his life so far. By reading and discussing stories that cover a wide-ranging field of different subjects, people come face to face with the flaws in themselves and in others. When I read about the man who fell passionately in love with a younger woman, I quickly lost sympathy for him as soon as he started searching for a new lover for his wife. Falling in love, okay. But trying, even if only in your thoughts, to shape the future life of the partner you plan to desert? No way! This was only a minor element in the story, but it highlighted a shadow in my own personality: an aversion to a thought or action that I wanted nothing to do with, not even in fiction.

I was amazed that I had reacted so strongly in my thoughts. At first, I could not understand why my response was so emotional. But this is typical of our shadow side: a deeply hidden side of our persona that can produce unexpected and inexplicable outbursts when challenged.

If you are part of a reading group or duo, you will eventually (and inevitably) encounter the shadow side of your psychological make-up. This shadow begins to emerge within the experience space created by the story, but in keeping with the scenario developed by the author and not in keeping with your own mental likes and dislikes. If this were not the case, you would never allow the thoughts or feelings that so offend you into your mind, so that you would never come into contact with your shadow side. The writer draws you into the theme that confronts you with your own mental, emotional or moral boundaries and exposes them to the harsh spotlight of examination, often in a manner that is more complex and more detailed than you would wish.

And then comes the magical moment: the break in the reading, which gives you the opportunity to say what is on your mind, whilst at the same time discovering that someone else has a completely different view and is not offended by the story at all! This simply means that the theme evokes fewer shadows in their psyche than it does in yours.

By hearing different responses to the same story – one forgiving and the other disapproving, one amused and the other deeply moved – your own psychological mechanisms are activated in the virtual space inside your head. It is there, in the shared experience with your fellow readers, that you learn. With no pressure or compulsion. With none of the linear expectations of therapy in terms of 'progress' or 'insight'. There is no need to agree with any of these interpretations. There is no need to judge anyone for holding alternative interpretations. You don't even need to find a 'solution' relating to the theme that is causing you so much trouble. All that happens is that you are given the opportunity to experience that the theme, about which your own thinking is so rigid, is capable of being looked at in a different way. This automatically makes your mental-emotional room for manoeuvre more flexible than it was previously and less hindered by prejudiced preconceptions and fixed patterns of thinking. By experiencing that your forbidden thoughts have a right to exist, you create for yourself more mental space and bring added flexibility into your life.

Moreover, it is not just shadows that are brought to the surface by the variety of themes within the texts. Experiences that people for whatever reason are not able to enjoy in the real world can be enjoyed in the virtual world of the imagination. For example, the world of people who are sick or are in need of care is often drastically reduced in size, so that there is frequently insufficient space for them to experience some important aspects of life. Perhaps they are not physically able to travel or seldom come into contact with other people and contexts.

The reading of stories and poems brings a wide range of possible experiences within the reach of these people; experiences that often transcend the boundaries of culture and time. For a person who has a preconceived view of, say, Muslim or African culture but has never had (or ever will have) the chance to meet people from those cultures, reading a literary text may allow him to discover that such cultures are actually rich and varied. In this way, via the experience space of his imagination, he gains a different and more balanced view of a part of the world that is physically inaccessible to him. No matter how limited someone's physical boundaries might be as a result of illness or disability, Shared Reading has the potential to take him anywhere he wishes.

An associative process

This broadening of people's horizons, achieved through reading or listening to a cycle of stories and poems embracing a variety of different themes, is hugely beneficial. It is not even necessary to deliberately compile the cycle in such a way that you hope it will cover all the required shadow areas. It is impossible for reading companions to draw up reading programmes that touch on every aspect of human existence! Besides, no one can know in advance which sentence or which aspects of a text will cause someone either to lose interest or to gain insight. In other words, the growth pathways of the participants can neither be predicted nor controlled. On the contrary, reading groups are free spaces for growth. The groups certainly create the necessary favourable conditions – a layered text, opportunities for the exchange of opinions, the freedom to speak (or not), an atmosphere of mutual respect and attention – but beyond that the process cannot be managed or directed. In the mental-emotional space created by the story the participants follow associative paths rather than rationally imposed routes. The author paints a powerful picture that is capable of generating numerous different emotions amongst the readers-listeners and leaves plenty of room for the use of their imagination. They are free to feel whatever they like about the text, without the need to justify this rationally and irrespective of whether or not the author explicitly intended to explore the theme in question.

By selecting a broad spectrum of texts, the reading companions give people the chance to share experiences and gain insights at a time and a tempo that is right for them. Without pressure and – hopefully – with a great deal of reading enjoyment.

Tips for practice

'Stories cannot break down boundaries, but they can drill holes in mental walls. And through those holes we can catch a glimpse of others, and sometimes we even like what we see.'

Elif Shafak

1. Plan to include a number of breaks in the story or poem you are reading. Check in advance to see where might be a good moment to pause. This could be at the end of a passage that will make your listeners curious about how the story continues, or at a point when a new character is introduced or does something remarkable, or where the use of language is particularly striking, etc.
2. Ask open questions that leave space for the participants to formulate their own reactions to the text. For example: 'What do you remember most about this fragment?'; 'What does this text do to you?'; 'Do you recognise this personage/situation?'.
3. Remain neutral and stay in the background. As the reading companion, your role is to stimulate conversation and keep open the space that makes this possible. If different opinions emerge within the group, you must never choose sides. Give everyone's opinion a right to exist, without judgement.
4. If you are a therapist in daily life, make sure that you don't slip into this role during the reading sessions. These sessions are not therapy and demand of the reading companion a much more reserved approach towards the participant than is common in therapeutic settings.
5. At the appropriate moment, bring the break to a close and refocus the participants' attention on the story or poem.

Give them enough time to formulate their thoughts but resume reading before their discussions wander too far away from the essence of the text.

6 Choose a varied selection of stories and poems for your series of reading sessions. Do not simply pick themes that you think will relate closely to the participants' living environment but also pick subjects that potentially seem remote for them.

3
Harvesting

The boy smiled, and continued digging. Half an hour later, his shovel hit something solid. An hour later, he had before him a chest of Spanish gold coins. There were also precious stones, gold masks adorned with red and white feathers, and stone statues embedded with jewels. The spoils of a conquest that the country had long ago forgotten, and that some conquistador had failed to tell his children about.

Fragment from: The Alchemist *by Paulo Coelho*

A time to harvest: gathering what you have rightly earned

Growth cannot be unlimited. Every upwards movement eventually reaches a phase where it evolves towards balance and completeness. A child grows up and becomes an adult. The grain ripens and a tree's blossom is transformed into fruit. At the end of a warm summer, it is time to bring in the harvest. The results of our labour and growth become visible and can be gathered in, so that they can be used for our further nourishment and enjoyment. In a material sense, we are paid for the hard work we have done, but at an emotional level we are also rewarded with a variety of new and pleasurable experiences, such as recognition, honour, attention, appreciation, warmth, joy and tenderness.

For people receiving care this is by no means self-evident, but even in their circumstances there is still a time to harvest. Someone who has recovered from a serious illness has every reason to celebrate and can be proud of what he or she has achieved, often as a result of great determination and patience. A child with a physical limitation who has difficulties learning how to sit or walk deserves all our applause. A patient who gains insight into the underlying patterns of his depression or burnout as a result of a therapeutic process has every right to reflect with satisfaction on his resulting growth in awareness and self-knowledge.

In a psychological context harvesting is about allowing new insights to take root in yourself. What you have achieved in terms of inner growth must now be given a place in your being. New experiences, images and ideas are installed inside your head and henceforth form part of your life's baggage.

We do not always give ourselves the time and attention we need. Harvesting is a culturally charged phenomenon that is subject to many different norms and prejudices. Some people like to harvest and frequently do it to excess, often at the cost of other people, organisations and the environment. They are not concerned about anyone or anything but themselves and simply wish to gather as much as they can. Others find it much harder to accept their right to compensation or rewards for their effort. They are afraid to ask for money for their work and pass this off as 'doing a favour for a friend', whereas inside they are unhappy because they have once again not been given the appreciation they feel they deserve. Or they let someone else take the credit for a success that was rightly theirs, simply because they do not want to be the centre of attention.

People who do not have the courage to harvest will continue to give without receiving until they are completely empty or become dissatisfied about themselves, because they fail to gain recognition from others. Whereas in reality that recognition is something that you must first be willing to give to yourself before you can get it from those around you.

Appropriate harvesting is harvesting the correct amount of recognition in relation to what you have done or achieved: not too much, but not too little either. In part, this is a matter of self-esteem. If you have done something good, take the credit and recognition that you have earned. Allow yourself to reap the rewards of your effort, whether those rewards be financial, material or emotional. People with a low sense of self-esteem often find it difficult to harvest as they should.

If you do it properly, harvesting is something pleasurable. It is a bit like enjoying the last sunny days of the year from the comfort of your back garden: a period of personal expansion followed by a phase in which you sample and savour the good things that life has given you.

For people receiving care, harvesting is a dimension to which extra attention needs to be paid. A stay in a hospital or a care centre is not generally something festive or agreeable. Someone who has recovered from a serious illness usually wants nothing more than to get back to their normal daily way of life as quickly as possible. Even so, it is important for care receivers to also allow themselves some time and space to enjoy the fruits of their labours and to celebrate the experience of growth and recovery. Even seemingly minor triumphs deserve to be recognised.

Harvesting is not only about securing a result or a reward, but also about keeping what you have secured. Whoever gains new insights but then fails to give those insights a proper and permanent place in their life will quickly lose an inner expansion of self that was within their grasp. People who have achieved a great deal in financial or material terms but then need to make superhuman efforts to maintain that level of success will usually end up burning themselves out. So only harvest what you have earned, seeking a good balance between giving and receiving. Allow yourself the 'luxury' of enjoying the progress you have made and make sure that you can retain what you have worked so hard to achieve.

As a care provider, the important thing in this phase is to assist your care receivers to harvest where they can, helping them to find new strength and insight from the growth and expansion that they have experienced. Shared Reading supports this process in a calm, relaxing and pleasant manner, which give its participants all the freedom they need to harvest their just desserts at their own speed and in keeping with their own capacity.

The harvest of Shared Reading

Shared Reading allows people to harvest at different levels. At the mental and emotional level, people experience an expansion of their range of options: the participants integrate the new insights they have obtained through their discussions with their fellow readers and see more possibilities for doing things differently in their lives. In addition, they are able to experience an abundance of new perspectives on human existence and on the world, as well as gaining a new understanding of different cultures and the past. This can give people a greater sense of nuance, by allowing them to see that their own problems and concerns are universal. The pleasant and safe atmosphere of the reading group (or reading duo) makes it easy to give the participants access to new growth and learning opportunities. By expanding the number of perspectives, insights and possibilities that people experience in this manner, it becomes possible for them to harvest the power within their own being.

Shared Reading also has great societal value. It is a low-threshold and socially acceptable activity that can have a therapeutic effect and contributes to a culture of social awareness and concern for each other.

Increased possibilities

By reading powerful literary texts and discussing them with their fellow readers, the mental and emotional worlds of the participants are significantly expanded, as we have already seen in the previous chapter.

This growth brings new insights. During the harvesting process, these insights 'land' and take root in the participants' minds, where they become integrated into their thoughts and behaviour, finding expression as a whole new range of opinions and perspectives that make them stronger and more flexible as people. The fact that someone is capable after reading a powerful story of giving a frustrating situation over which he has no control a place in his life, without breaking down, results in a strengthening of that person's ability to cope. Similarly, the fact that someone can show new understanding of behaviour that he would immediately have condemned in the past results in a strengthening of that person's empathy.

If someone grants themselves the necessary time and space to give these insights a place and allows them to take root in his mind, not only will his manner of being change, but also (in due course) his manner of doing. A person who discovers through discussion of a story that his own viewpoint is simply one of a whole variety of possible viewpoints will be able to harvest a new degree of emotional flexibility, as a result of which he will also be able to see new possibilities for behaving differently in his life. Instead of continuing, for example, to tolerate his difficult relationship with his partner, with all the anguish this entails, he now understands that other options are possible: discussing the situation calmly; confronting his partner with some home truths; breaking off the relationship; admitting the possibility of falling in love with someone else; forgiving the partner for an act of infidelity… Whereas in the past this person would have approached the situation with unbending rigidity, he is now able to harvest a new flexibility in his thinking and feeling. In a similar way, someone else who has recently lost a loved one can learn through reading and discussing a story that there are different ways to respond to death other than inconsolable grief. New alternatives magically open up: a route of gratitude, a path of inspiration, a road of remembrance and reflection… This person also harvests an expansion of his emotional flexibility and freedom.

By allowing the insights obtained through Shared Reading into their lives, the participants are able to harvest new possibilities that had previously been denied to them and a far greater and much freer space in which to explore those possibilities. It is as if they have been dealt a new hand of cards, with which they can approach and deal with life in a new and different way. By embracing this expansion of mental and emotional space in their being, they become stronger and often more assertive. Whereas before they were restricted to a limited number of rigid routes in their mind, they can now see a dazzling range of new options. New vistas are opened up in their thinking. People suddenly realise that they do have a choice and that they are capable of much more than the limitations imposed by their habitual patterns of behaviour.

And even if this expansion of possibilities does not lead to concrete changes in behaviour, the expansion process itself always remains beneficial. The people concerned may not yet be different on the outside, but they are already different on the inside. They have become people who in their thoughts at least now dare to consider alternative pathways for reaching their familiar destinations. Or perhaps they might find the courage to aim for a new destination altogether. One thing is certain: having the thought is the first crucial step towards eventually taking positive action.

Seeing the universal in the personal

By reading texts about the most disparate range of themes, personages and events, the participants in Shared Reading discover that the things that are causing them problems are actually quite common. They realise that others – not only the fictional characters in stories but also their fellow readers with whom they discuss those stories – also have positive and negative experiences in their lives, not to mention strange thoughts, lurid fantasies and even hormonally inspired outbursts! Whereas in the past a person might have thought that he was alone with his weird ideas and opinions, literature shows him that this is not the case. There is nothing we can feel or think that has not been felt and thought before. No matter how bizarre, deviant or rare our personal hatred, rage or sexual frustration, someone somewhere has already been there. This is a liberating realisation, which gives people the opportunity to find peace in their inner world.

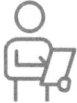 'The reading aloud did me good. It made me feel better, because we had the chance to say what we thought about it during the breaks.
It is interesting to know what others think. You can weigh your own opinions against theirs, which allows you to think that maybe you are not so abnormal! You know that you have a place in this life after all! If you follow the reading closely and understand it, you can forget most of the modern nonsense that is blocking your mind.
This helped me a lot during my depression. You get the idea: They are just people like me! For me, this was like a revelation. I am just the same as them! I can recognise myself in other members of the reading group, and also in the stories we read.'

Frans, participant in a reading group for psychologically vulnerable people

During a series of reading sessions the texts will deal with various cultures and different periods of history. Sometimes the author will be from your own country; sometimes the story will come from an unknown and more exotic land; sometimes the text will be new; sometimes it will be hundreds of years old; the reading might even be a piece of poetry. Whatever their origin and nature, all these texts reveal themes and problems that are recognisably universal. Consequently, people discover that the difficulties they face are not new, but have been experienced in all times and all places; that a mother in Syria grieves no more (and no differently) for her lost child than a mother in Flanders; that people in the 18th century wrestled with the same hopes, fears and uncertainties about the meaning of life and death as you and I today; that Shakespeare and Goethe described with the same depth of nuance the emotions we all experience in our day-to-day lives, even if their use of language is more formal and sounds strange to our ears. This results in a feeling of connection and also offers a sense of perspective.

As we begin to see universal patterns in texts from other times and cultures, we feel greater connection with the people from those periods and places. We experience the richness of history and cultural diversity, which is brought to life so vividly in the words of the stories and poems.

As a result, our preconceptions and prejudices gradually begin to disappear. Someone who, as a matter of habit, never has anything good to say about 'foreigners' might suddenly discover during a Shared Reading session that Africa has a fascinating and centuries-old tradition of storytelling or that a writer from Iran can express perfectly the complexities of the problem with which he is also struggling. This develops a degree of sympathy and understanding for other cultures.

By reading literary texts from other traditions that express a different philosophy of life, it is possible for us to escape from our preoccupation with our own 'superior' way of doing things, a tendency to which our Western culture is particularly prone. This allows us to gradually free ourselves from our fossilised patterns of thought, which we have often acquired through our education and upbringing. Someone who comes from a socialist or Catholic background will often be imbued with ideas and opinions that reflect that background. By reading texts that challenge these ideas and opinions and then discussing the resulting implications with other people who come from a different background, we are encouraged to see our own viewpoint from a different perspective and to be more open to creativity in all its many different forms. This leads in turn to the realisation that we are nothing more than a brief footnote in the pages of history, which creates a strong bond of solidarity with the countless millions who have gone before us. As a result, we think less in terms of 'us' and 'them', identifying instead with the universal elements that we can see in the most diverse range of texts.

To be, or not to be, that is the question:
Whether 'tis nobler in the mind to suffer
The slings and arrows of outrageous fortune,
Or to take arms against a sea of troubles
And by opposing end them. To die, to sleep,
No more; and by a sleep to say we end
The heart-ache and the thousand natural shocks
That flesh is heir to: 'tis a consummation
Devoutly to be wish'd. To die, to sleep;
To sleep, perchance to dream – ay, there's the rub:
For in that sleep of death what dreams may come,
When we have shuffled off this mortal coil,
Must give us pause—there's the respect
That makes calamity of so long life.
For who would bear the whips and scorns of time,
Th'oppressor's wrong, the proud man's contumely,
The pangs of dispriz'd love, the law's delay,
The insolence of office, and the spurns
That patient merit of th'unworthy takes,
When he himself might his quietus make
With a bare bodkin? Who would fardels bear,
To grunt and sweat under a weary life,
But that the dread of something after death,
The undiscovere'd country, from whose bourn
No traveller returns, puzzles the will,
And makes us rather bear those ills we have
Than fly to others that we know not of?
Thus conscience does make cowards of us all.

Fragment from Hamlet *by William Shakespeare*

Safety

Much of what people harvest from Shared Reading has little to do directly with their way of thinking, but is more concerned with what might be called the 'gut feeling' of pleasure, satisfaction and security that it gives them. This, too, is valuable and healing, because it provides gratification at a basic level that is often felt more powerfully than thinking.

By reading in groups, the participants are given a sense of belonging, of being connected with others. Reading groups are sociable, even convivial, but there is also a feeling of solidarity with people in general, irrespective of when, where and how they lived. This contact with others in the broadest sense gives a warm dimension to Shared Reading. The pleasure that the participants derive not only from shared reading, but also from listening together and discussing together in a pressure-free environment, is often heart-warming. A simple nod of agreement when a particular passage is read or the sharing of a moment of humour is often enough to create a bond, without the need for many words. In short: Shared Reading generates a relaxed atmosphere that is experienced by the participants as being pleasurable in a way that is almost tangible: the pleasure of being in the same boat as everyone else and enjoying something that enriches both yourself and your fellow readers.

Shared Reading also gives people who do not normally read the chance to come into contact with serious literature. Some people never read at home; perhaps because they don't enjoy it, or don't have the time, or find it too difficult. Yet the experience of reading and discussing powerful stories and poems in the company of others can be massively empowering.

This was certainly the case for Anke, a dyslexic ergotherapy student, who was highly intelligent but found her studies difficult. Because of her disorder, she always felt that reading was not something for her – until she was persuaded to take part in a Shared Reading session and a whole new world opened up for her. The experience that reading can be enjoyable and that you can simply step into the world of the author's imagination came as a revelation to her.

Rina suffered brain damage as a result of a car accident. Consequently, she is no longer able to read a book by herself without the use of various complex aids. She even finds it too difficult to follow an electronic reading assistant. However, she is more than able to participate in a Shared Reading group, which gives her the opportunity to once again experience the pleasure of taking part in stories without difficulty.

Amina, a young woman with autism, also finds it hard to read at home, but loves to attend the reading group at her local day-activity centre:

> 'Shared Reading is fantastic. Our group is small, but we have lots of fun. This puts me at ease. I am not good with crowds and I wouldn't be able to take part in a large group. The voice of the reader is also pleasant and calm.
>
> I almost never read at home. I sometimes look at the newspaper or at the advertising bumph, but that's about all. In the evening I am too tired to read, but in the reading group you make the necessary time. I would never do that at home. I am too busy keeping the house clean and with hundreds of other things. I just never get around to reading. In the reading group, I never find it a problem to concentrate. You can just listen to the stories and the different opinions that people have about them.'
>
> *Amina, participant in a reading group for psychologically vulnerable people*

It is striking how many people are loyal when it comes to regularly attending their reading sessions. Even if they do not often take an active part in the discussions, they keep on coming back time after time, simply because they experience the sessions as enjoyable and/or beneficial, even if they sometimes find it hard to explain why. I can remember one woman exactly like this. She never joined in with the exchanges of opinions, but simply followed what the others said. One day, when an external visitor asked the participants about their reasons for taking part in Shared Reading, this woman answered: 'I have been coming to this reading group for three years, and that says all that needs to be said.' And that was, indeed, all that she said – but it made clear that the sessions held great value for her.

Much the same applies to the the reading companions. Most of them are unpaid volunteers, but very few fall by the wayside. This shows that Shared Reading is interesting for them as well. Reading aloud in a group or with an individual reading partner is a form of care, but one which offers a good balance between giving and receiving.

Transfer: the reading companion as a parent figure

> There were eleven of us. Eleven small boys, the sons of my father. Eleven boys, each with a handkerchief in his pocket.
>
> Our house had long walls and there was a weeping willow in the middle of the garden. Old.
>
> Twilight was approaching. Grandfather began his evening walk in the dark shadow of the wall. At the same moment, we all went and sat under the willow. Just like we did every evening.
>
> My father rolled out the carpet under the tree. He sat down and rested his back against the trunk. We sat on our haunches around him and he began to tell us a story.
>
> 'There was magic in his poems.' That was the opening sentence of the story.
> We knew that it was a story about grandfather's father. The father of the father of our father.
>
> 'He was the poet of his people,' continued my father. 'And he was against the father of the father of the shah.'

We looked at grandfather. He was leaning on his walking stick, listening.

(…)

When the story was over, grandfather walked to the tap to wash his handkerchief.
He washed his handkerchief and hung it on the branch of the weeping willow to dry. Just like he did every evening.
At the same time, my father stood up. He rolled up the carpet and leant it against the trunk of the tree. Following this, he went across to the tap to freshen up. And then it was our turn. We all ran to the tap and splashed water on our hot faces. To dry ourselves, we pulled out our small handkerchiefs. Finally, we ran back to the tree to hang them among the branches. Two of theirs and eleven of ours.

We discussed it with each other. We had to.
'But father? What happened to those poems?'
'They live on in the thoughts of people,' my father replied.
'And the magic? Did it die? Did it disappear as well?'
'No. The magic could never die.'
'So where is it now?'
'Perhaps in the fingertips of one of you.'

The darkness crept up behind us and took our house in its embrace. We searched for signs of the magic in our fingertips. The wind played with the handkerchiefs on the branch. With the onset of the dark, fear crawled under our skin. Unannounced, the full moon appeared. And it gave us great comfort.

Fragment from: And then it was our turn *by Kader Abdolah*

The reading companion who supervises the Shared Reading session reads the story or poem aloud in a calm manner in a pleasing and comfortably arranged room. This automatically evokes memories of the participants' childhood or youth, when they were also read to in a relaxed setting: a mother or father who read a story at bedtime; a school teacher who read a story in class. Most people had this experience of being read to when they were young. As a result, this creates a psychological transfer: unconsciously, the participants associate the reading companion with the parent or teacher of yesteryear. In the chapter on 'Growing' we saw that mirror neurons work more effectively in interaction with someone from your own group than with an outsider. This same principle applies during the Shared Reading sessions. If someone reads you a story, you automatically give that person a position within the group that is closest to you personally; namely, your original family. In other words, the reader becomes – to some extent, at least, and whether you like it or not – your mother or father. For this reason, the listeners during Shared Reading sessions quickly bring all the emotions they feel about their parents into the mental-emotional space that they now occupy as a result of listening to the story. In this way, the reading companion becomes a kind of archetypical parent and evokes a number of emotions that the participants felt about their own parents.

This means that during Shared Reading the participants automatically find themselves in a psychotherapeutic situation that is comfortable and safe. The reading companion reads them someone else's story – the story of the author of the text – in the secure environment of a pseudo-parent-child relationship. These associations with the participants' personal history quickly create an 'aha!' moment, a moment when something clicks inside their head and they suddenly gain insight. When this happens, their own story becomes merged with the story that is being read. If I am angry at a married man who falls in love with a younger woman during the story, I need to ask myself whether this reaction has something to do with my original family and the way in which I relate to my father and mother. Mental connections of this kind generate powerful emotions and can lead to numerous therapeutic insights and experiences, without any formal therapeutic practices being applied.

This principle works equally effectively even when people have had a poor relationship with a father or mother. Because they are being read to, they unconsciously see the reader as a surrogate parent figure. When that person reads aloud to them in a warm and encouraging manner, the listeners quickly position the reader in their mind as an idealised parent. In this way, the listeners can bring what they lacked from their parents in the past into the story, whilst at the same time experiencing what it feels like to have a warm and committed (surrogate) parent, even if their relationship with their natural parents was very different and even if they were never read to as a child. This is one of the reasons (amongst others) why carers specialised in youth rehabilitation work or youth psychiatry like to collaborate with Shared Reading. With young people, this transfer process works even faster than with adults. But even with adults it is important for the reading companion to create a warm and comforting atmosphere.

By experiencing this archetypical structure of the parental role in a safe and reassuring environment, the participants in the reading session absorb the content of the story much better and are therefore much more easily able to experience learning and growth. This opens up a broad pathway in their memory along which recollections from their childhood, which would otherwise be much less accessible, can now emerge. If you are asked to talk about something that happened when you were four or five years old, you will probably have to dig very deep in your memory. But if someone reads to you in pleasant and relaxing surroundings, very concrete memories about a moment when you were read to as a child will almost certainly emerge, often complete with details about the person, place and book in question.

In older cultures there frequently were storytellers who told the stories of their nation or people and passed on the great events from their history by word of mouth. Powerful narratives were handed down from generation to generation, always in the same way and without changing anything.

This oral tradition has largely been lost in our Western culture. We no longer tell the stories of our history to each other, as a result of which we feel a less strong connection with our cultural roots. Social cohesion in countries that still have a strong storytelling tradition, as is often the case in Islamic and African cultures, is much greater. Shared Reading repairs and regenerates something of that social solidarity, in part by the very process of reading aloud, but also in part – and more importantly – by discussing what is read.

'Today, I read the story about *Frog and Tortoise* to a group of people with mental difficulties. It was about the plants that grow in the garden. To visualise the theme, I brought along some real seeds and allowed the participants to plant them in a pot on the table. At the end of the reading session, I took out a plant I had previously placed under the same table, which I gave to the group to look after. They promised me that they would take good care of it.

Some of the people in this group use a computer to help them communicate. This slows down the storytelling, but at least ensures that everyone is involved in the reading process. A young man from another reading group came along with me, supposedly "to keep an eye on me", but it was clear that secretly he enjoyed the reading.

As usual, I printed off a copy of the story for everyone, which they were allowed to take home afterwards for re-reading. For the clients in this group I am very clearly "the storyteller" who comes to read to them. If I later meet some of them in a different setting, they immediately start talking to me about the stories we have read together. They only know me as "the reader".

Ivo, therapist and reading companion in a care facility for people with limitations

Strength

The integration of new insights and possibilities, combined with the experience of a feeling of warmth and security, makes it possible for the participants to draw new strength from Shared Reading sessions. They suddenly realise that they have more space in which to move and are capable of far more than they ever thought. This experience of a new spaciousness is empowering. It gives people a clearer and more complete picture of who they are and they learn that in addition to their weaker side – which is often painfully obvious for people who are dependent on care – they also have a stronger side. They now feel that they have a place, a right to belong and exist, and this notwithstanding their imperfections and inner peculiarities, which are often much more universal and much more 'human' than they imagine. Little by little, they stand more securely in life, more aware of who they are and what they can do. In short, they have a better appreciation of their own value as a person.

Stories help people to find this new strength, because they also shed light on aspects of life that are flawed and incomplete. Good stories are seldom about perfect harmony or people that possess ideal qualities. On the contrary, they often show the worst side of human nature, the dark and hidden side that is full of bad thoughts, bad feelings and bad habits. But they also show that these things are normal and okay. Even people with very bleak personal histories often take part in Shared Reading, because it allows them to find points of contact with their own lives in a manner that gives them new energy and resilience.

'The stories that most affect me stay locked in my memory. During the week I might suddenly be reminded of them by a similarity with something that happens in my life, and that strengthens me.'

'The stories come back to me quite often. If I hear or see something, sometimes I think: "That's how it was in the story."'

Frans and Amina, participants in a reading group
for psychologically vulnerable people

At first sight, this harvesting of greater mental resilience and new strength does not always seem spectacular. But even small changes can be indicative of a significant increase in self-confidence and self-esteem. The key thing is to be aware of what is going on inside the participants' heads and to see what Shared Reading is doing to them and for them. This is illustrated by the testimony of Eva, who supervises a reading group in a psychiatric care home.

'We are reading *Everything Arranged* by the Dutch author Thomas Verbogt. The evening before, I re-read the story. Some parts of it make me laugh out loud. But in the reading group the next day everything remains quiet, apart from the occasional snoring of one of our less attentive participants. "That woman who looks as though she knitted herself?" asks Emiel. "What exactly does she look like?" Lieven then chips in: "I think it's an odd text. The main character behaves so strangely."

I am surprised by these reactions. Far too often I assume that if I think something is funny or moving, others will think the same. Lieven also surprises me with his honesty. When I started

86   SHARED READING

reading here at the end of last year, the residents always said that everything we read was "good". Happily, that has now changed.

We talk about what songs we would like at our funerals. Emiel doesn't need much time to think: *Sophietje*, a 1965 song by Johnny Lion. He begins hesitantly to sing and the others join in: "She drank lemonade through a straw, my Sophietje, on a terrace in Amsterdam..." Sven would like something from Bach's *Matthew Passion*, while Eric prefers *My Way* by Sinatra. "At my funeral," says Lieven, "I would like to have the Mass in Latin, like it was when I was a child."

Meanwhile, lunchtime has arrived. I have noticed a change here, too: the listeners and those who read along now remain attentive until the very end of the session. In the past, those whose task it was to set the table kept on looking anxiously at the clock, afraid that they would be late for duty. Perhaps I have become calmer when reading?

Sadly, we don't have time to read a poem. Even so, Lieven lends me a book of poems by the Flemish author Gaston Durnez. The reading moments in this psychiatric care home are becoming more and more genuinely Shared Reading. That is good and it makes me feel good, as well.'

Eva, reading companion

Building blocks for a caring society

Shared Reading not only enriches the lives of the participants but also offers a significant added value to society as a whole. It generates important impulses for greater human connectivity and social solidarity. In an age where loneliness has become a societal epidemic, this is more than welcome.

A reading group that is active over a longer period is a strong building block on which to erect a more caring society, simply because the people in the group learn how to care for each other. They are cocooned in the warm, safe and protective ambiance created by the layering of the text and the relaxed nature of the setting, in which they can enjoy listening to a story and then discuss it without feeling the need to defend a particular point of view. This slow, quiet and pressure-free atmosphere makes possible a number of learning moments, as a result of which the participants are not only able to gain insight from each other but also mirror concern for each other.

The participants treat their fellow readers and the author who reveals himself in the story with great care. Even if a particular text holds less appeal for them or fails to reflect their opinions, they never criticise the author. Instead, during the discussion of the texts the participants experience that different opinions and different tastes have a right to exist alongside each other, without the need to try and 'win the argument' or to paint the author in a negative light.

Shared Reading helps to form and strengthen a culture of community; a culture founded on the basis of stories that are repeatedly told. By reflecting on these stories, the participants build up a coherent mode of behaviour that is regarded as 'good' and 'acceptable' within this culture. Any group that exists for any length of time will also gradually build up shared values. In a reading group these values include empathy, affection, connection, solidarity, a sense of belonging without the need to prove yourself, respect for other opinions, and patience. The participants can learn and practice the values in question by listening together to the stories and poems, reading along with them, and discussing them afterwards. Moreover, by reading texts from world literature people come into contact with the values of different cultures. Their mirror neurons cause them to reflect on these things and to acquire understanding and respect for them. As a result, a communal spirit is gradually developed by the members of the reading group, not only towards each other, but also towards the wider outside world.

There are also numerous opportunities for mirroring care and for learning from this reflective process in one-on-one reading sessions. The experience of being given individual attention in a pleasant and informal atmosphere and the possibility to be heard and to respectfully exchange thoughts about all your worries and emotions with the reading companion is something that many people will not have known since childhood. They take this experience with them into their daily lives, where a ripple effect can develop in many different ways. One possibility, for example, is that they start to read to their own children, partner or sick relative. Alternatively, they might consciously give more genuine attention to others in their environment.

> 'Once when I was reading to a group of people in a rehabilitation centre, one of the participants had no personal relationships at all. He had drunk himself into complete isolation and had lost all his family. He had no friends who were not alcoholics like himself.
>
> One day, he was suddenly surprised by a line in a short story by George Saunders: "There will still be moments of good companionship". After he had read the line, he touched the page and stroked the words with his fingers. "Yes, that is true," he said. The story was about an old man who wanted to die and the drunkard was able to see his own life reflected all too clearly in the text. When he spoke about "moments of good companionship", I knew that he was referring to the other people in the reading group, by whom he was surrounded in the room.
>
> Until then, he had never read anything aloud in the group – he was a difficult character – but that moment of revelation, when he stroked the page and repeated the words, changed everything. From then on, he began to read regularly for others, in the growing conviction that moments of good companionship would indeed still come…'
>
> *Jane Davis, founder of The Reader organisation*

Powerful therapeutic effects without high costs

Shared Reading has a significant therapeutic effect without the costs usually associated with classic therapy. For people in a vulnerable situation, who often need to spend a large part of their budget on medical or other care, reading is an easily accessible activity that supports their psychological well-being in a relaxed and easy manner without them having to pay fees they could otherwise not afford. Following a long-term trajectory with a psychologist or psychiatrist is not always possible or appropriate for everyone, often if only for financial reasons. People with limited financial resources frequently scrimp and save on things that do not directly contribute towards their material subsistence, whereas psychological care can actually be life-saving for someone in a precarious mental position. A reading group or reading duo can serve as an anchor point that offers people the opportunity to grow in a pleasant and safe environment, providing them with relaxing and healing experiences, but without putting them under financial pressure. For the participants, Shared Reading is wholly free of charge.

Moreover, reading is a socially acceptable activity. There is no shame or stigma attached to telling people that you belong to a reading group, whereas it is often more difficult to explain that you are undergoing therapy with a psychologist or psychiatrist. In other words, the social threshold for Shared Reading is low.

Also low, both for society in general and for care institutions in particular, are the costs associated with Shared Reading. The reading companions are either external volunteers who agree to work for a particular care facility or else are employees of that facility who run the sessions during their normal working hours. The preparatory training of the reading companions – the cost of which is usually paid by the facility where the person in question will later read – is recommended, but is not expensive. Apart from providing a pleasing space for the sessions, perhaps with some tea, coffee and biscuits, no other infrastructure or resources are required. In comparison with the societal investment involved in training psychologists and psychiatrists and the subsequent cost of providing psychotherapy, Shared Reading offers a low-threshold method that can achieve sustainable effects in terms of inner growth and resilience with only a minimal budget.

The necessary conditions for harvesting

Slowness and serenity

Just as the harvest is brought in from the land during the last calm days of summer, so the process of harvesting from Shared Reading also demands an atmosphere of slowness and serenity. The discussions during the breaks in the reading sessions can be animated and intense, but to bring the most meaningful aspects to the surface it is essential to offer the participants the necessary time and space for reflection.

When you listen to someone who reads at a steady speed, you soon find yourself relaxing. Your breathing becomes calmer and your thoughts become less agitated and more ordered. Sometimes you may even find yourself falling into a kind of soothing trance, in which you just float along on the stream of words. This sense of slowness and serenity makes listeners more receptive to the content of the text. As a result, the discussions during the breaks in the reading also acquire a different quality and depth of meaning than is the case in a purely intellectual discussion. Shared Reading is not concerned with an intellectual or literary analysis of the text, where the focus is on the skill and originality of the different arguments put forward. Shared Reading is all about 'sampling' the text and letting its contents sink slowly into your mind; about enjoying the experience of being read to; about reflecting on what you have heard and allowing new insights and ideas to rise to the surface of your consciousness.

'The best way to read a text aloud? Not everyone can do it. You need a slow and soft voice, like a singer's, without stumbling over your words. A voice that has a soothing influence on people's mood. That is how I can best get into a story, because if you read a story together, you need to be able to let it sink in before you can understand it. That is why it is necessary for the reader to read slowly, because the content of the text needs digesting. Sometimes a story reminds you of similar circumstances in your own life and then you drift away on your dreams for a few moments, so that you lose the thread of the next part of the story. You then need to jump back in and push what you have just been thinking to the back of your mind. This process is repeated frequently, so that you constantly move in and out of the story. But the slowness of the reading means that you never become completely lost.'

Frans, participant in a reading group for psychologically vulnerable people

It is possible for silences to occur in the mid-reading discussions, without any need to immediately fill them. This gives the participants the possibility to think things over for themselves. What are their opinions about the text and the themes, characters and events it contains? For this reason, it is important for the reading companion to allow sufficient time during the reading breaks for the conversation to develop spontaneously. If he immediately asks a question, it is likely that only the most extrovert and self-confident participants will reply, so that they will end up dominating the conversation. By allowing a pause in which nothing is said, everyone is given the opportunity to develop their own thoughts and emotions about the text in the quiet of their own head.

This brief initial period of focused calm significantly improves the quality of the discussions during reading breaks. The role of the reading companion in this respect is subtle but oh so important. By also positioning himself in the same energy field of focused attention, he makes this energy available for the entire group. In short, the reading companion becomes an energy anchor point; he holds open the space in which a deep and safe discussion is possible. By remaining neutral and in the background, he gives the participants the chance to go more deeply into their thoughts and emotions, allowing them to give these things a place, so that they can harvest and learn from them. In total calm and security, they are able to explore what they truly think about the text and how they feel about the alternative interpretations put forward by the other participants.

In essence, this is not so very different from what usually happens in a normal therapeutic conversation with an individual. In such a conversation the therapist will also deal carefully with whatever issues emerge and will give the client the necessary time to order his thoughts and emotions. The main difference is that the moments of silence that fall in a one-to-one therapeutic session seem much more threatening to the client, or at least more stressful. Why? Because there is no one else in the therapeutic space who can break that silence. In group therapy sessions silence has a different and more anticipatory quality, since group therapy is a more targeted process. In that case, silence means waiting for what comes next, so that the conversation can continue.

When silence falls in a reading group, all those present briefly relax. It is a moment of calm, without the expectation that anyone will respond to it. This kind of silence can be liberating and gives everyone the chance to recover their inner composure.

For this reason, when silences naturally occur during reading breaks it can sometimes be beneficial to let them continue for a short while. This mental pause often stimulates someone from the group to reflect and to formulate a new idea about what has been read, so that the conversation resumes organically. The reading companion needs to be able to sense the difference between an uneasy silence that is lasting far too long and a fruitful silence, where fresh thoughts are being developed that still need a little extra time for ripening before they can be spoken out loud.

By allowing moments of silence and by connecting with the group participants within that silence, it may not seem as though the reading companion is actually doing very much, but in reality he is subtly making it possible for the participants to harvest, without steering or directing them in any way.

In reading duos, where the reading companion reads aloud for a single person, the same dynamic is also at work. Once again, the silence and the companion's focused attention are of great value for the listener. This is clear from the testimony of Lien, who took part in a project where medical students read to cancer patients.

'I go to my first reading session in the haematology department with mixed feelings. On the one hand, I am curious and keen to get to know my reading partner. On the other hand, I am worried and a little afraid. What if it doesn't click between us? What if I can't find the right words? I enter the reading room with my heart in my mouth. I introduce myself hesitantly and offer to pour us a cup of coffee. From a practical point of view, a good way to avoid getting thirsty and dry-mouthed during the next half hour; figuratively, a gesture of warmth and affection. In short, a good opener for any session.

I tentatively try a first question: 'How are you feeling?' In some ways, it seems a stupid question, because I already know the answer. A patient with leukaemia can only be feeling bad. But my intuition tells me I still have to ask the question. The answer is no surprise, but immediately makes a deep impression on me. It is soon clear from a number of things my reading partner says that she is currently in a very bad place.

Although my bookcase is packed with books about cancer, her mood affects me deeply. She gives the disease a face; scientific knowledge is transformed into a real, live patient, sitting in front of me. Even so, I am glad I asked that first question, because I get the sense that it does my reading partner good to be able to talk about her difficulties.

Once the introductions are over, I start reading our very first text together. Occasionally, I stop and inquire about her thoughts and feelings about what has been read. I try to get a conversation going but the lack of familiarity between us is still too great.

A week later, I try again; this time with a completely different text. To my relief, things are more relaxed. And the following week there is still further improvement. The atmosphere is more open and for the first time I get the feeling that I can actually mean something to my reading partner. The story that I read brings various emotions to the surface. One aspect in particular is painfully familiar to her and causes her to stop and reflect on the seriousness of her illness and the many difficulties she has had to face since that first hard diagnosis. These thoughts make her cry.

My first reaction was one of panic: *Oh no, this is not what I expected! How should I react? Should I say something? Surely I must try to break this uneasy silence? But how? I can't possibly say that I understand her pain, because I don't. How can a carefree nineteen-year-old student say that she understands what a terrible disease like acute leukaemia does to a person? But I have to find something to break this silence. Don't I?*

But the right words won't come and so the silence persists for what seems like an eternity. After thinking long and hard, the best I can arrive at is: 'It must be very difficult for you'. After that, my reading partner continues her story. She takes the time to ventilate her feelings, to get things off her chest. She explains how she tries to stay positive, but freely admits that it is not always possible. It is hard to hear the people around her constantly saying 'It will be all right in the end', when she herself has serious doubts about the likely outcome. The fear of dying flits daily through her thoughts like an unwelcome guest.

> The only thing I do while she is telling her story is listen. I say nothing. It is only when a new silence is reached that I say: 'I think it is very brave that you try to remain so positive and I truly hope that you manage to overcome your illness.' Not perhaps the most eloquent response, but at least it comes from the heart.
>
> As I leave, she thanks me. She says that the session has done her some good and that she enjoys having the opportunity to tell someone what she is really thinking and feeling. At first, I don't understand what she has to thank me for. I hardly said a word in the half hour we were together! But later I realise something that I already unconsciously knew. In reality, it is not necessary to give an answer for everything. Sometimes silence is the only answer and in many cases this is all the patient really needs.'
>
> Lien, medical student

Give the participants the freedom they need

'To every thing there is a season, and a time to every purpose under the heaven. A time to be born, and a time to die; a time to plant, and a time to harvest that which is planted.'

Ecclesiastes, 3:1-2

The harvesting and expansion of mental space in Shared Reading does not always take place in neatly defined phases. Often, these things are part of a dynamic that involves a rapid succession of events: people start to read and listen to a story; they break through the barriers of their familiar thinking and feeling; they harvest the insights that result from this; they let go of their old ideas; they find peace in a new balance. This cycle can sometimes repeat itself more than once in a single reading session.

The circle does not necessarily need to be made complete. For example, during a phase of growing insight, it is possible that a moment of reflection will follow, after which the reader once again gets carried away by the excitement of the continuing story. Sometimes it is only after a number of reading sessions that the accumulated insights of the previous weeks suddenly begin to fall into place.

Sooner or later, however, a point is reached when the person in question or the people around him start to notice that he is changing; that he has more mental room to manoeuvre; that he has become stronger and more firmly rooted in life. As a reading companion or caregiver, it is important to take account of this change, but without projecting any expectations in terms of possible growth or greater insight onto the participants. Whatever happens, happens – and it makes no difference whether it happens quickly or slowly. That is one of the strengths of Shared Reading: the freedom it gives people to participate at their own speed and with the level of commitment that feels most appropriate for each individual. People who want to say something about the text and what it makes them feel are free to do so. People who want to just sit and listen are free to do that as well, safe in the knowledge that no one will challenge their right to be silent. Nobody is ever asked directly what he or she thinks about the text, because this would take away the participant's freedom to take part in the reading session without conditions or obligations.

It is important that reading companions do not try to harvest things on behalf of their participants. It is not the companion's task to interpret or frame what someone says about a particular text. This is one of the main differences with therapy: the insights that arise spontaneously in the participants are not intentionally analysed. The great value of the conversations and discussions that develop during Shared Reading is precisely that they enable the participants to discover their own insights and adjust their perspectives accordingly, without being explicitly 'guided' in a particular direction by someone else. Other members of the group may occasionally do this, but the reading companion must resist the temptation at all costs. It is not his or her task to act as a therapist.

Of course, when it is clear that someone is finding things difficult during a conversation or discussion, it is perfectly normal for the reading companion to give that person some attention. This does not always need to be expressed in words; sometimes a quick glance or a brief confirmatory nod of the head is enough to show that the reading companion is aware of what the person is going through. It is also a good idea at the end of each session to check that everyone is feeling okay and has recovered from the emotional impact of the session before returning to their home or room.

The human dimension remains crucial when supervising a Shared Reading session, but it needs to be repeated that there is a major difference with therapy. By allowing the participants the necessary time and the freedom to develop and frame their own insights, they experience that they are capable of achieving their own mental broadening and deepening, without anyone else guiding them or trying to explain what they are thinking and feeling. This enhances their emotional resilience and strengthens their self-image.

Tips for practice

'That is what literature offers – a language powerful enough to say how it is. It isn't a hiding place. It is a finding place.'

Jeanette Winterson

1. Read the text calmly and at a steady pace, without adding too much of your own interpretation. Resist the temptation to act.
2. At the start of a break in the reading, allow a brief moment of quiet before you ask your first question. This gives the participants time to shift their focus from the text to their own thoughts and emotions in response to its contents.
3. Don't be afraid to also allow pauses and moments of silence during the subsequent conversations and discussions.
4. Facilitate the conversations and discussions, but without directing or interpreting their content. Look for connections between the thoughts and experiences of the different participants, so that the exchange of views becomes something more than a series of loose fragments.

4
Learning

The Lake Isle of Innisfree

I will arise and go now, and go to Innisfree,
And a small cabin build there, of clay and wattles made;
Nine bean-rows will I have there, a hive for the honey-bee,
And live alone in the bee-loud glade.

And I shall have some peace there, for peace comes dropping slow,
Dropping from the veils of the morning to where the cricket sings;
There midnight's all a glimmer, and noon a purple glow,
And evening full of the linnet's wings.

I will arise and go now, for always night and day
I hear lake water lapping with low sounds by the shore;
While I stand on the roadway, or on the pavements grey,
I hear it in the deep heart's core.

William Butler Yeats

Sifting and letting go

Once the harvest has been gathered, you need to do something with it. A farmer who harvests the crops from his field sells them and then evaluates whether or not the harvest has been a good one. Will he grow the same things again next year or will he try something else? Has all his hard work and effort been sufficiently rewarded? Or should he, perhaps, switch to different crops?

People who are in need of care do not always realise that they can also gain new insights from the care experience. Most care recipients have the tendency to think 'I am what I am'. They accept their complex medical condition, their physical deficiencies, their depression and their vulnerability, assuming that this is how things will always be. They are locked in a stationary situation, from which they expect no further change. As a result, they no longer attempt to alter that situation or do anything other than what they are familiar with.

Caregivers can play an important role within this context. Helping people to learn is an integral part of providing good care. By looking behind us and learning from the experiences of our past, we become wiser and more solidly rooted in life, which allows us to see our way forwards more clearly in the future. If a caregiver can assist his patient or client in this process, it represents an important step in breaking through the negative 'I-am-what-I-am' mentality.

Although we often assume the contrary, learning is not the same as absorbing and storing different kinds of information. A man can have a whole library full of books and a three terabyte external hard drive on which he saves the mass of information he gleans from the internet, but unless he does something with all this knowledge it will bring him no benefit.

Just as binge eating has nothing to do with proper nutrition, so the storage of information for information's sake has nothing to do with proper learning. If you binge eat, your body only stores the nutrition it needs and disposes of the rest as ballast. And it is the same with learning:

your mind only stores the information it needs to make sense of your knowledge and experience. Everything that cannot be used for this purpose should be jettisoned.

Letting go is an essential part of learning. It involves a calm assessment of everything that has happened to you and an analysis of the insights you have gained as a result, on the basis of which you then decide what you want to keep in your life and what you no longer need. You sift through all the information, knowledge and experience you have gained, classifying it in order of importance. You retain the things that are still meaningful for you. You let go of the things that have become superfluous.

This is only possible if you take sufficient time for the necessary processes of reflection and introspection. You need to ask yourself – and understand – why some things are important to you, and others are not. Just as in nature the energy of trees turns inwards as autumn progresses, shedding their leaves in preparation for the winter, so it is similarly beneficial for us humans if a period of expansion, growth and harvesting is followed by a calmer period for taking stock of recent developments. Where have I come from? Where am I now? What have I learned? What can I let go? What things should I carry with me for the rest of my journey?

We can also learn from emotional events in the same way. These phases of learning are important, since they allow us to grow and prevent us from falling time after time into the same familiar patterns of behaviour. For example, a blazing row with someone is often followed by a moment of calm, during which we are able to harvest an increased level of assertiveness, because we have had the courage to express and defend our opinion, which makes us feel stronger.

Even so, we need to be on our guard. After a period of emotional intensity, there is always a strong temptation to try and get back to 'normal' as quickly as possible. Which is fine… until the next conflict arises, either with the same person or with someone else. If, however, you pause for a moment of reflection after a fierce emotional encounter of this kind, you may perhaps come to the insight that these repeated conflicts are draining energy from both sides. If you are not careful, this may lead to an irreparable breakdown in your relationship.

This insight can lead to a change of behaviour. The next time a conflict arises, instead of reacting forcefully perhaps you will be more inclined to take a step back, so that you can calmly reflect on what is happening and explore the reasons behind it. In this way, you may be able to see more clearly your own part in causing these repeated conflicts and moderate your behaviour accordingly. As a result, the stormy conflicts of the past now lead to a moment of learning, which persuades you that in future it will be wiser to deal with others in a less aggressive and more constructive manner.

Clearing the clutter from your mind

Shared Reading also creates space for moments of reflection, learning and letting go. During a reading session, people can acquire many different kinds of insight that allow them to reset their perspectives. This can result either from their own response to the contents of the text or from their exchanges of opinion and interaction with others in the group. In particular, this interaction often leads to a nuancing of their own 'black-and-white' judgements, so that their thinking becomes more open and broad-minded. If they are able to integrate all these insights and experiences by taking the time to give them a proper place in their being, a new phase of learning will be possible. This, in turn, will make it possible to let go of old opinions about yourself and others, freeing your mind of old patterns of thinking and fossilised emotions that are no longer appropriate for the larger and more flexible mental-emotional space that you now possess.

Countless stories and poems contain elements that can help readers and listeners to learn from their own experiences and to let go of things that are hindering their growth. Many people are unable to achieve this for themselves. They are often trapped in situations from which they cannot escape without the stimulation of literature to assist them. For example, someone might find it impossible to come to terms with their grief for a lost loved one. But if they listen to a story in which one of the characters dies and then discuss this with their fellow readers, they might eventually come to the insight that death is an inevitable part of life, which may make it easier to finally let go of the lost loved one.

Likewise, old convictions, a negative self-image, a negative opinion about others or about life in general are also things that can become rusted in your mind. If you continually worry about the same problems over and over again, your thoughts will be constantly occupied by their negativity, which prevents you from being able to learn. It is only when you can let go of those thoughts that your thinking and feeling will be able to move forwards, so that you will once again find the peace and calm you need to reflect and arrive at deeper insights.

Many Shared Reading companions have commented on the fact that the participants often see things in literary texts that they themselves failed to see, or at least interpreted differently. This is something that I experienced at first hand during the reading session with the story of *Judith* by Charles Ducal, where it became clear that many different interpretations of the love-sick father's behaviour were possible. I might have found his actions reprehensible, but others thought they were amusing, endearing or even caring. This taught me that my own thinking on this and a number of other matters was perhaps too black-and-white, whereas I had previously regarded myself as someone who was balanced in my approach to my own life and the lives of others. I saw that maybe it was time to let go of this idealised self-image and start being more flexible in my opinions.

In other words, Shared Reading soon disabuses you of the notion that you know it all. Similarly, it also shows you that you are not alone with your problems. Since ancient times, great literature has been wrestling with themes that are still highly relevant for many individuals today. This sense of 'not being the only one' helps people to let go of their stress, freeing them from their conviction that some problems are so personal and so all-consuming that you have to sacrifice your entire peace of mind on the altar of their importance. Sometimes these 'problems' can be seemingly banal. For example, a man who works ridiculously hard, so that he can have a house that is bigger and better than his neighbour's. This is vitally important to him, so much so that it forms the basis for his entire identity. In contrast, many literary stories deal with personages who attempt to form their identity based on interior rather than exterior characteristics: on what they have learned, on the extent to which they are able to understand and empathise with what happens in life, on their ability to inspire and connect with others, on their capacity to make the best of their talents and strengths… Identities of this kind are determined by inner drivers, and not by what a person owns in material terms. Reading about such things can be highly instructive and change-inducing for many people; perhaps even for our house-obsessed friend mentioned above!

In this way, Shared Reading helps you to clear all the useless clutter from your mind. By reading stories and poems with a wide range of themes and personages and by discussing personal baggage, they put behind them the injuries and fixations of the past. If, for example, someone was regularly beaten as a child and has built up his identity around the idea of 'I am weak and hurt', Shared Reading might slowly help him to realise that his history in reality reveals him to be someone with great resilience, who instead of being weak is actually very strong. As a result, his focus shifts from the harm that has been done to him in his life and switches to the fact that, in spite of everything, he has survived. This makes it possible for him to build up a new identity based on a new foundation of 'toughness', an underpinning that is every bit as valid as 'vulnerability', but probably much more useful.

In short, Shared Reading not only offers people the possibility to rid themselves of redundant patterns of emotional behaviour (such as revenge, fear, jealousy, etc.) in a relaxed and creative manner, but also helps them to let go of their former attachment to their pain and feelings of hurt.

'I drew a line…'

I drew a line:
this far, and no further,
never will I go further than this.

When I went further,
I drew a new line,
and then another line.

The sun was shining
and everywhere I saw people,
hurried and serious,
and everyone was drawing a line,
everyone went further.

By Toon Tellegen
Translated by Judith Wilkinson

Letting go and keeping hold of fragments: dementia

The process of letting go takes an extreme form in people with dementia, even though in this case the letting go is largely unconscious. Gradually, but sometimes with a sudden increase in pace, the sufferers of this condition let go of the contents of their memory. Memories fade, the recognition of people becomes more difficult, the command of language weakens, and the functions of everyday objects become a mystery to them.

Throughout this process of letting go and loss, people cling tightly to precious bits and pieces of their mind. They repeatedly tell the same stories, which are often memories from when they were young. If you ask someone with dementia what they were doing an hour ago, they will not be able to tell you. But if you ask them about their best friends from primary school, there is a good chance that you will be told the same story a number of times, often with a clear recollection of details.

Stories, especially old stories, remain fixed in the human memory for a long time, even if a great deal of other information and practical knowledge disappears. This illustrates what the Dutch media and cultural researcher Frank Hakemulder says about the structure of memory and the function played by stories:

Stories are so powerful precisely because the human memory has a narrative structure. Our memory consists of a series of things we have been told. Some of these things have their origin in the stories we hear or see. In short, human life is interwoven with stories.[3]

This explains why Shared Reading is also so worthwhile for people with dementia. Often, they have lost contact with yesterday, but can still recover numerous isolated incidents from their library of memories. Stories and poems that they knew during their youth often spark off a glimpse of recognition. By taking them back through the texts of their younger years, fragments of memory from that period of their lives can be triggered, so that through association they sometimes tell part of their own story. In addition, people with dementia enjoy as much as anyone else the pleasure of being read to and discussing what they have heard. What's more, the texts do not always have to be texts from their youth. Perhaps surprisingly, contemporary texts can also stimulate a response.

As with people in other care contexts, the text is a catalyst to talk about things that otherwise might never have spontaneously been mentioned. This is clear from the testimony of Lisa, who works in a residential care centre and regularly reads for residents with dementia.

3   https://lezerscollectief.be/wp-content/uploads/2020/06/In-goed-gezelschap-Frank-Hakemulder.pdf.

'During the reading of *The Green Suitcase* by Diane Broeckhoven the reactions from the group come thick and fast. "Oh dear!" says Vera, referring to the bossy friend of the main character. "I'd soon get rid of her!" Vera laughs, and the group laughs with her. "Imagine having to put up with someone like that all the time," adds Linda. "Not me!"

In the meantime, Annie looks across at her friend Elsa. It almost seems as if she is checking that Elsa is still awake. Elsa nods and smiles back at her. These two ladies both prefer to follow the story in silence, although sometimes they endorse what others say and laugh along with the rest of the group. True, Elsa does occasionally nod off, but when I call her name and ask if she is okay, she usually replies: "I'm just resting my eyes, but I am still listening!"

Irene looks constantly at the others with a surprised expression on her face, as if she wants to emphasise that the story is exciting. She frequently confirms this by saying "It's a good story", but during the subsequent discussions she often drifts away and starts talking about herself to the resident sitting next to her. At moments like that, perhaps she is no longer with us or no longer understands what is happening.

Most of the residents look at me when I am reading aloud, although there are three who keep their eyes lowered. These three seldom react to the story, but at least they regularly laugh along with the group.

Vera laughs loudly and looks around. She is searching for reactions amongst the others. "I thought something like that would happen," she says when the friend in the story starts throwing everything around.

"That's not nice; that's naughty. No, not nice," says Lutgarde.

Evelyne nods. She often agrees with what others say.

At the end of the story, it is once again Vera who pipes up: "Finished already? But I want to know what happened after that!"

With poetry the reactions are different. There I sometimes find that my own interpretations can help the residents to share their opinions and experiences. Sometimes I also give them a copy of a poem, so that they can read it again back in their room. I know that some of them won't bother, but that doesn't matter.

During a poetry moment for some of the residents in an advanced state of dementia, we read some verses by the Flemish poet Alice Nahon and Dutch cabaret artist Toon Hermans. I read very slowly and repeat some of the lines. When I come to the words "It is good to look into your own heart", it is nice to see how most of the residents still know how the verse continues. As they say the words, most of them have a smile on their face. Because it is something recognisable? To me, at this moment they seem fully engaged in the here and now and they seem to understand what is going on. True, after the reading there are fewer reactions than in the other group, but at least they have all followed what I have been saying closely.

For our reading sessions, we meet together in the living room. There is a comfortable atmosphere, with few other stimuli or distractions. After a while, Dora reacts to the text. "That's difficult," she says. "I'll need more time to think about that." Poetry can indeed be difficult for our residents and so I give them the time they need. Yet even Klara, who is often restless and generally prefers to wander around, talking to herself, is listening attentively and seems to be enjoying herself. Anna thinks about her strict mother and says that she will get a smack "if I don't understand it properly". Eline smiles and says: "Not anymore, you won't".

After an hour, I notice that the attention of the residents is starting to drift and that it is time to stop. At least for today.'

Lisa, caregiver and reading companion
in a residential care centre

Shared mental-emotional space as a learning space

Learning is not something that you do alone. During Shared Reading sessions, it is certainly the case that the discussion moments in between the readings are a huge stimulus for the learning process. In the chapter on 'Growing' I referred to the mental-emotional space that is expanded by Shared Reading. In part, this expansion is generated by the layered nature of the text, in which the author develops themes in a manner that goes beyond our ordinary, everyday thinking. But in part it is also due to the opportunity to talk about and discuss these themes, which makes it possible to see that other people have other opinions and interpretations. It is by mirroring the contents of the text and each other's reactions to those contents that our inner space is enlarged.

But it goes much further than that. We do not remain alone in our enlarged inner space. We share that space with others, so that we create a common or shared mental-emotional space in which we can learn about each other's different perspectives. We each build up our own mental-emotional space in a different way. For example, a person with a generally pessimistic view on life will construct his space differently from a person who is more optimistically minded. Unless you know someone very well, you will usually not know how their mental-emotional space has been constructed and therefore what preconceived ideas are locked inside this person's head. When you both listen to the same story, you will both imagine a different version of that story. Sometimes these versions resemble each other; sometimes they are light years apart.

When a story contains largely factual events, there is little room for divergence. Someone who falls from a horse will land on the ground. That will look the same inside everyone's head. But when events are more emotionally or morally charged – for example, when someone cheats his neighbour – this makes it possible for more variation in people's responses. One listener might think that the character in the story was fully justified in his actions because he needs to protect his family against his neighbour's aggressive behaviour. Another might think that such dishonesty cannot be justified in any circumstances.

Strongly layered stories in which different outcomes, meanings and metaphors are possible in turn make possible different interpretations. By listening to this kind of story in a group (or duo), different participants are affected by a wide range of different experiences and images. Everyone imagines inside his own head a version of the story that largely contains the same elements, but which has a completely different look and feel.

When the participants discuss the story and exchange with each other the thoughts and emotions it generated within them, they open up their own mental-emotional space for outside input. While I regard the love-sick father as being overly aggressive, my neighbour in the group might see him as being charmingly romantic, while a third person might be reminded of someone he knew in his youth who was exactly the same. In short, we invite our fellow readers to step into our own mental world, as a result of which everyone's mirror neurons are activated by what they hear, see and feel.

Through this complex exchange of perspectives, we learn to correct and add nuance to our own way of thinking. In this way, our mental-emotional space becomes a learning space for others. And vice versa.

Neuroplasticity: flexible brains

Learning is something we can do throughout our life. In our modern society, we often assume that people are the way they are because they were born that way. As a result, we further assume that they cannot change. If they couldn't do something in the past, they will never be able to do it in the future. So what is the point of trying to teach them? In much the same way, people receiving care are not always given the room they need to grow. They are all too quickly written off as being too weak, too old or too damaged to learn anything new. But in reality our brains are remarkably well suited to making adjustments. Growth and expansion is always possible, even when we are adults. Perhaps the change process is less smooth and less fast than when we were children, but it can still take place.

Our brain cells are formed into a supple matter, which changes as our life progresses. The technical term to describe this is neuroplasticity. We are all born with a huge surplus of brain cells. During our development as children, we use some of these cells a great deal and others not very much, depending on the kind of environment in which we grow up.

In Europe, for example, we have much less need for an ability to find water than people living in the bone-dry heartland of Australia. Consequently, our brain cells and the neurological connections that are necessary for us to smell, see and sense water have become atrophied. Because the human brain requires large amounts of energy to operate, it deals efficiently with the synapses that are less frequently used. It is almost as if it locks them away in some kind of cerebral cold storage. If the circumstances in our life change, so that these synapses suddenly become necessary – let us imagine that climate change turns Europe into a desert – they are removed from our mental 'fridge' and reconnected. As a result, before too long we will be able to identify the best and wettest place in our garden to sink a well. This is an example of neuroplasticity: the suppleness of the brain to adapt to new circumstances.

Neuroplasticity is activated whenever we learn something; for example, a new skill like riding a bike, driving a car or speaking a foreign language. Initially, our brain is not capable of performing these tasks, but with practice over time we are soon able to master them. Via fMRI, it is possible to see how the brain activates the new neurological connections that are required to make this feasible.

Similarly, after brain damage it is possible to see how certain functions within the brain are relocated. If, for example, someone has suffered from a cerebral haemorrhage resulting in trauma to the area of the brain where the motoric control of the right arm is located, so that the limb can no longer be moved, brain scans have revealed that the adjacent zones in the brain are increasingly activated during the recovery process. As a result, the arm's motoric function can be repaired much more effectively than might originally have seemed the case. This mechanism also explains why someone who suddenly becomes blind quickly develops an improved sense of touch, which makes it possible for them to read braille, even at an advanced age. The same enhancement applies equally to the senses of sound and smell, and even to the power of imagination.

The same processes are also at work in the mental-emotional domain, so that we can practise how to react in ways that are different from our normal patterns of behaviour. For example, fighter pilots are trained how to remain calm in the most stressful conditions, so that they can continue to act responsibly for the greater good. This is not an inborn quality, which would mean that you have either got it or you haven't, but is a skill that can be learnt.

In other words, by stimulating our neuroplasticity we can continually experience more and thereby continually expand our mental-emotional space. This occurs whenever our brain cells are triggered to follow new pathways, which is possible in many different ways: by learning new behaviour and doing new things; by seeking out new environmental stimuli; by exploring new modes and patterns of thought; and by experiencing new emotions.

Ideally, the development of new patterns of thought and behaviour requires a model. And for this purpose, Shared Reading is ideal. By repeatedly reading new stories and poems, the participants come into contact with a multiplicity of new experiences and different environments. One week you read about a love affair in a country village; the next week you read about a murder in the desert. Each story gives you new environmental stimuli and previously unknown experiences. Via your mirror neurons, you are able to invite the world of the story inside your head.

In this respect, the mid-break discussions relating to the text are particularly useful. One person can be angry at the behaviour of a personage in the story, while someone else understands that behaviour better and is more forgiving. For the angry reader, the mildness of his fellow reader is perhaps a reaction pattern that he has forgotten in his own life. By reflecting on this mildness and empathising with it, he re-opens a neural pathway in his brain that has not been used for some time. Instead of thinking 'I am always strict about these things; that is just the way I am', he now tests out an alternative option in his head. In much the same way, a person who has a fear of other cultures may discover through reading *The Thousand and One Nights* that the Islamic tradition contains many wonderful stories. Perhaps this might persuade him to start looking differently at his Arab neighbours, who until now he has avoided. Another example? Someone whose only response to opposition is aggression (verbal and physical) or flight may realise through reading different literary texts that there are other ways to deal with conflict situations, such as talking about them or resolving them calmly by making firm decisions.

Opening or re-opening pathways in the brain is one thing; whether the person concerned will continue to use them is something else entirely. It remains a matter of free choice. Perhaps the angry man and the cultural xenophobe will only experience the potential benefits of an alternative course of action just once, before returning to their old habits. But at least the door to a new form of reaction has been opened, even if only briefly. A learning process has been initiated and it is up to the individual to decide whether or not he wishes to pursue it further in his daily life. The option is there, if he wants it.

Thanks to neuroplasticity, we have the ability to learn and change until relatively late in life. We can continue to expand our mental-emotional space. This is the space that is described in powerful terms by the authors of literary texts. Within this space, we can step into a world of imagination and experience things for which we previously had no model; for example, a world where even the magical is possible.

Through his realistic, tangible and sensory descriptions of this world, the author has the power to take us there, time after time.

Viewed in these terms, the experience of Shared Reading involves a series of learning moments, during both the reading of the texts and the subsequent discussion of their content. The reading sessions create an experimental space for new thoughts, ideas and possibilities. The multiplicity of options that this allows the participants to explore ultimately leads to a greater plasticity in their personalities. That is how they can learn and grow.

It is important for caregivers and reading companions to give the people in their charge this all-important opportunity to grow. It would be wrong, for example, to assume that some texts are 'too difficult' for certain kinds of participants. Even men and women who are not used to reading 'serious literature' can have fascinating and mind-opening discussions about its contents. Simply talking about these things, even if you don't fully understand them, can have a beneficial effect. In this context, it is important that the reading companion should avoid giving information about the author, the place of his work in literary history or his stylistic peculiarities. In Shared Reading, the focus should be exclusively on the experience and perception of the participants, with the text as the starting point and the finishing point of everything.

> 'We often found it surprising that our reading companion chose such difficult texts, written by serious authors. In short, real literature. When that happened, we thought: "Good for you!"
>
> Riet, head of a daytime activity centre for psychologically vulnerable people

No obligation to learn

'Poetry heals the wounds that reason inflicts.'

Novalis

I have mentioned it already: one of the great strengths of Shared Reading is the freedom it gives to the participants and the absence of any predetermined expectations. This expresses itself in the manner in which the participants learn. In Shared Reading this happens much more freely and much more spontaneously than in educational or therapeutic contexts.

Classic forms of learning take as their starting point a clearly defined and carefully prepared learning plan, with a set of specific objectives about what the pupil or student must know at the end of the trajectory. Learning plans of this kind are rational and structured, with clearly defined steps that must lead progressively towards the learning objectives, with intermediary evaluations being held along the way, so that remedial action can be taken, if there is a risk that the objective will not be met quickly enough or fully enough.

The situation in care environments is comparable. Therapies are developed around a number of objectives or at least have the intention to move the client in a particular direction that is deemed to be beneficial. For example, an occupational therapist can set clear milestones for a child, which makes it possible to see how that child's learning evolution is progressing. Similarly, a psychotherapist will ensure that during his sessions with a client he frequently refers back to the basic theme for which that client is receiving counselling. If someone's fundamental problem is indecisiveness, then during a session that discusses, say, one of the client's sick relations, the therapist will also make the connection with the client's underlying lack of resolution to clarify the client's ambivalent attitude towards that relation. Occasionally, the therapist will also check to see whether the client is gaining insight into the basic causes of his problem and will ask him what specific and concrete action he plans to take to bring change into those areas of his life where he is currently experiencing difficulty. The client will often resist this probing and attempt to avoid the therapist's seemingly confrontational questions. Usually, he will not be inclined to deal actively with the core issues, because he knows that this will be far from easy.

With Shared Reading, the participants are spared this uncomfortable probing. There are no objectives and no predetermined intentions. Even so, the reading sessions offer space and numerous opportunities for learning in a manner that is both free and unpredictable. In a reading group, there is no question of a learning plan or of a cleverly contrived sequence of texts. As I have already made clear, it is impossible to know in advance which parts of a text will trigger a response in one of the participants, so that he can achieve insight or a broadening of his thinking and/or feeling. For this reason, it is not necessary to compile a series of texts designed to highlight a specific theme. On the contrary, the texts should be as open and as varied as they can be, so that they will automatically contain a large number of impulses, often seemingly insignificant, that can spark off a reaction that might lead to learning and growth.

Because the learning space is deliberately left open, each participant is able to extract from the text and its subsequent discussion the things that are important for him, and not the things that the reading companion perhaps expected him to extract. For example, during the reading of the story *Powdered Snow* by Tobias Wolff, which I mentioned in the chapter on 'Growing', not everyone in the session caught on to the fact that the father had surreptitiously called the police to draw them away from the barrier on the closed road, so that he could slip through unnoticed. It was only when one of the participants explicitly pointed this out during the discussion that the penny finally dropped. Yet even though they had 'missed' this key aspect of the story, many of them still enjoyed the visual description of the snow-covered landscape through which the father had driven with such skill and shared the feeling of the main character that 'I am safe with my father in this car'. For this latter group, it was the image of the father as a strong and reliable man that was important, whereas the group who had seen through his trick tended to see him as an untrustworthy rogue. Each participant chose the elements of the story that were useful and interesting for him, based on his own experience, his attitude and the way in which his mental-emotional space is coloured.

The reading companion made no attempt to steer this process. There was no criticism of those who had failed to catch on to the father's trick, nor praise for those who had understood it immediately. In short, there is no 'right' or 'wrong' interpretation. There is only what the individual participants regard as important to them.

True, during the subsequent discussion of the text it is possible that some people's initial interpretations may be modified, but this happens in a free and spontaneous manner. And that is what makes Shared Reading so fascinating: people are given the freedom to decide for themselves what they want to learn. Or what they don't want to learn. Sometimes a text simply has no appeal for some of the participants, and that is fine. It is never the intention to keep digging in the text until everyone eventually finds something to which he can relate. 'This text does nothing for me' is a reaction every bit as valid as 'This text has shaken me to the core'. Both can exist alongside each other, without being judged by the reading companion and the other participants.

This freedom inherent in Shared Reading reduces people's reserve and resistance towards reading. There are no 'musts'. Everything is possible; nothing is forced. There is no expectation that the participants will draw insightful conclusions from the story that will allow them to make improving changes in their everyday life, which is often the assumption behind a therapy session. It is perfectly possible that useful conclusions may be drawn, but this happens spontaneously, without the need for the participants to be guided in a particular direction by the questions of the reading companion. The participants allow themselves to be surprised – and sometimes overwhelmed – by the theme of the story or poem and by the clever way in which the author has developed it. This stimulates thoughts and insights to come to the surface that might otherwise never have been consciously considered if the same theme had been discussed in an objective-based therapy session.

This spontaneous amazement, in combination with the session's relaxed atmosphere, creates breathing space. People discover almost by accident the hidden corners of the rooms of their mind, corners they would otherwise never think to clean out. The safe environment of the reading group makes them more willing to make connections between the text and their own lives in ways that can be applied in their day-to-day reality.

Having said that, the learning process in Shared Reading is not completely unstructured. The freer aspects of the process take place within a framework that has a number of recognisable elements: the session starts and ends at a fixed time; usually, both a short story and a poem are read; the reading companion plans three or four breaks for discussion; the poem is read twice, discussed, and then read again.

This structure lends a degree of calm and predictability to the reading sessions. It is the conduit through which the participant's free flow of thoughts and ideas can pass. But the discussion of these thoughts and ideas is not endless; at some point, the reading companion will always bring the participants back to the text. As a result, learning emerges from a combination of the session's serene structure and the freedom that makes it possible for each participant to explore his personal mental-emotional space in an unstructured manner, reflecting on the text and on what others have to say.

By exchanging their experiences of the text as perceived from their individual backgrounds and by listening to each other respectfully, the participants give each other the precious gifts of learning and growth, without there being any question of therapy. Shared Reading does not work in the same focused manner as therapy and pills, but it is potentially far more effective. Why? Because it teaches people a procedure from which they can benefit their whole life long. If someone is only treated with medication, at some point he will probably no longer need his pills and will stop taking them. But this has nothing to do with a learning process. Such a process has a longer-lasting effect and, as we have already seen, is cheaper and less complex than most forms of therapy.

Letting go of rigidity in care organisations

'We all have the tendency to walk in step. We need structures to organise our lives, but sometimes it is necessary to forget structure, if we want to build new mental bridges. It is by reading poetry and experiencing art that these new neurological bridges are made.
Art is not a pastime or something for 'out of hours' that is only found on the fringes of society. The artistic playground must be positioned at the centre of our society. It is the place where we create new possibilities.'

Maud Vanhauwaert, Flemish poet and performer

To a large extent, hospitals and other care systems and administrations are based on fixed – and sometimes overly rigid – procedures, which are focused on providing good and effective care to their patients and clients. Once these procedures have proven their worth, the care institutions are reluctant to let them go. Pressure from government to provide efficient care with limited resources reinforces this tendency. When budgets are tight, every decision needs to be weighed carefully. Of course, at one level this leads to operational stability and reliability, but there is also a risk that it will compromise the organisation's ability to continue learning. If things are done simply because that is what the procedure says must be done, without any form of critical (re-)assessment, there is a strong likelihood that the organisation's flow will eventually rust into rigidity.

For this reason, Shared Reading can benefit not only its care-needy participants but also care institutions and their employees. Caregivers can find it liberating to occasionally be released from the iron grip of procedures, enjoying instead the comparative freedom of the reading group. By experiencing for themselves the free and relaxed manner in which texts are read and discussed, they may also find themselves subject to a new dynamic that will allow them to grow, harvest and learn.

This can give them refreshing new insights, not only in their personal lives, but also in their professional lives and the way they deal with colleagues, clients and patients within the organisation.

In this sense, Shared Reading can even be seen as a form of team building. If care workers can experience in a safe and non-threatening context that different people read the same situation in different ways, this can only help to improve the interaction within and between teams. This has been confirmed by the testimonies of various teams in care facilities for psychologically vulnerable people, who took part in a research project investigating Shared Reading and its impact on care personnel.

'Our care centre took part in a research project to see if Shared Reading can have a supportive effect on teams working in an organisational context. Shared Reading as an HR initiative is a new idea, so little previous research had been done.

Working with two management trainees, I helped to set up a pilot study into the possible effect of Shared Reading on teams. More specifically, we looked at the effect on autonomy and self-direction within teams, on the development of trust between teams, and at the level of general satisfaction with meetings. However, we were also on the look-out for other possible effects that were not specified in advance.

A number of teams volunteered for the project, which involved taking part in a 30-minute Shared Reading session before their weekly team meeting, and this for a period of six weeks. During these sessions, the team members explored a diverse range of stories and poems by authors such as Arnold Lobel, Tommy Wieringa, Martinus Nijhoff and Philip Larkin. They followed the text as it was read aloud and then discussed its contents and their implications.

The effect of the sessions was charted in a series of questionnaires and interviews. The results suggested that Shared Reading had no effect on the pre-defined areas of interest – self-direction, trust between teams and satisfaction with meetings – but did generate other positive effects on the workfloor. The participants experienced greater openness in the communication between team members and found it easier to discuss things with their colleagues. They also thought that the sessions increased the feeling of connection and solidarity within the team, leading to a better overall atmosphere. Some even said that it was worth taking part in the sessions if only for the sense of calm and relaxation they experienced.'

Eva, HR manager

Similarly, Shared Reading with an individual person can also be a highly rewarding experience for a caregiver. This makes possible the development of a more personal relationship than in a reading group, so that the reading partner is increasingly regarded more as a person and less as a client or patient. This, too, generates a learning process. Stepping outside the formal caregiver-care receiver relationship can be a real eye-opener. This was what Lien discovered, when she took part in a project in which medical students read to cancer patients.

'The first few reading sessions were a bit awkward, but as the weeks passed we started to have some really good conversations. It wasn't all emotional stuff; there was also plenty of room for lighter moments. My reading partner used the stories I read to create new stories of her own, often based on memories of her past. Little by little, I saw a real person emerge from behind the facade of a woman whose dignity had been eroded by the terrible illness with which she was afflicted. This new image was the image of a wise and sophisticated woman, who carried with her a large rucksack filled with fascinating experiences and a true zest for life.

What I find most remarkable about Shared Reading is the way you can become "infected" with the emotions of your reading partner. When I saw how she brightened up when I read a particular passage of text, I soon felt a similar feeling of satisfaction, because I had the feeling that somehow, even if only in a very small way, I had been able to help my reading partner to escape from the hard reality of her life. It made me feel good to see how she blossomed when she began to talk about her children and how she laughed when she told me about funny incidents from her past. Her stories inspired me, touched me and, above all, made me empathise with her deeply.

Happily, my reading partner has now recovered. She only needs to come back to the hospital for check-ups, so we no longer see each other. On the one hand, I find this sad, because I enjoyed our reading sessions. On the other hand, I am grateful that I had the opportunity to take part in the project. It was a real rollercoaster of emotions, but it was unquestionably one of the most amazing things I have experienced so far in my young life.

I began the project as a naive student, someone who could fill books with her knowledge of the miraculous workings of the human body, but knew next to nothing about the thoughts and emotions of a person who suddenly discovers that those miraculous workings sometimes let us down. That is what Shared Reading has taught me.

I will take this experience with me as I continue to practise my profession and I am convinced that it will help me to become a better doctor in so many different ways. Shared Reading made me realise more than ever before that you should never reduce a patient to a set of symptoms and a schedule of treatment. Behind the broad clinical picture, a wide variety of thoughts and feelings are also at play.

Paying sufficient attention to these thoughts and feelings is just as important and just as healing as the medical treatment itself. What's more, you don't need any medical training to be able to do it. A little bit of empathy and a drop of the milk of human kindness is all you need – and that is what makes it so wonderful!'

Lien, medical student

Tips for practice

'That is what learning is. You suddenly understand something you have understood all your life, but in a new way.'

Doris Lessing

1. Choose a wide range of texts to read aloud. Don't be afraid to vary the authors, cultural origin, age, style, themes, etc. Do not underestimate your readers: even people without much formal education or who are psychologically vulnerable can cope with layered literary texts.
2. Allow the text to speak for itself. Do not give any background information about the author, his other works, his literary reputation, etc.
3. When discussing the text, ask open-ended questions.
4. Do not attempt to steer the discussion in any particular direction. Allow the participants to pick out the elements of the text and the discussions that are meaningful for them. Remember, however, to return to the text once the discussion has dragged on for too long or is leading nowhere.
5. Give the participants the necessary space to process the emotions and thoughts generated by the text and the discussion.
6. If there are participants who also wish to read aloud, allow them to do so. It makes no difference whether their reading is fluent or stumbling: their thoughts and emotions will always shine through in the sound of their voice. This makes it possible for them to contribute in an even more intense manner to the overall group experience.

5
Relaxing

Sometimes a-dropping from the sky
I heard the sky-lark sing;
Sometimes all little birds that are,
How they seemed to fill the sea and air
With their sweet jargoning!

And now 'twas like all instruments,
Now like a lonely flute;
And now it is an angel's song,
That makes the heavens be mute.

It ceased; yet still the sails made on
A pleasant noise till noon,
A noise like of a hidden brook
In the leafy month of June,
That to the sleeping woods all night
Singeth a quiet tune.

Till noon we quietly sailed on,
Yet never a breeze did breathe:
Slowly and smoothly went the ship,
Moved onward from beneath.

Under the keel nine fathom deep,
From the land of mist and snow,
The spirit slid: and it was he
That made the ship to go.
The sails at noon left off their tune,
And the ship stood still also.

Samuel Taylor Coleridge, Excerpt from
'The Rime of the Ancient Mariner'

Re-energising the depths of your being

Whoever is able to learn and to let go of what he no longer needs will be able to find a new calm and peace of mind. After all the many thoughts and emotions have passed fleetingly through your head, you let the things that really matter slowly sink into your being. This resting phase is essential if you want to achieve deepening and thereby come into contact with the true elements of your own self, the elements that (can) truly make the difference in your life. This takes you to the level of the great existential questions, the questions that are key to your identity as a person: 'Who am I and why do I do the things that I do? What is my life really about?' You will only be able to reflect deeply on these matters if you can first achieve the required degree of relaxation.

It is vital for caregivers to help their patients and clients to attain this relaxed state of mind. This does not mean keeping them as physically still as possible, if necessary through the use of medication, but rather helping them to find a mental calmness that will allow them to develop deep and meaningful new insights, on the basis of which they can make decisions that can be applied in their everyday lives. By rediscovering this mental serenity, they are able to see more clearly where they currently stand in life and where they want to go.

With the help of this of intense relaxation, people are able to re-energise the deepest parts of their being. This is very different from the image that many people have of 'relaxation'. For the majority of us, relaxation is about doing things: playing sport, meeting friends, visiting the cinema or a museum, etc. Slower variants include watching television or surfing on your computer. However, none of these activities are truly relaxing – they are all forms of being active and gathering information.

To re-energise your being, you need to make the necessary time for yourself, to slow things down until you find complete mental calm and quietness. You can compare it with nature. After the trees let go of their leaves in the autumn, they enter a state of rest during the winter. All their strength is directed inwards and the flow of sap is reduced. They rid themselves of everything they do not need to help them through the long, cold months of winter. But once this period is past, they burst back into life with the renewed vigour of spring. People also regularly need this same deepening period of total calm, a time for contemplation and reflection that will revitalise their being. It is during these periods that they find the strength to move forwards again.

If you are able to reflect with a totally relaxed mind, by the time your process of reflection comes to an end you will know precisely what you want to do. You will not yet have started to do it, but you will at least know where you want to go. And based on this clarity of thinking, you will be able to make the plans that will allow you to start your new journey. What's more, during this phase of deep calm, you will also develop the necessary willpower to carry out your plans. Willpower is not about pushing forward with all your might, but about finding clarity of direction, deciding consciously to move in that direction, and then finding the strength of purpose to carry that decision through. The period of calm reflection will have made it possible for you to recharge your batteries, so that you can now move forward again in a manner that is connected with your deepest self.

A society in overdrive

Society as a whole also regularly undergoes the cycle I have described in this book: starting new initiatives, allowing them to grow, harvesting the results, drawing relevant lessons from the experience, reflecting on those lessons in moments of deep calm, before finally moving forward again and implementing what has been learnt in practice.

That, at least, is the ideal scenario. In reality, the phases of learning and reflection are often omitted in our fast-moving modern world. As a society, we are overly focused on starting, growing and harvesting. Unfortunately, once the harvest has been gathered, we seldom stop to reflect inwardly in all serenity on what we have learnt from our experience and to see what important things we wish to retain and what irrelevant things we wish to relinquish before continuing our journey.

There are countless examples of this. Companies often start new projects that they are able to grow successfully. But once they have harvested the profit, they immediately seek to invest it in a new project that will bring an even greater return. In this way, they remain constantly focused on expansion and growth, without ever stopping to think about the good and less good aspects of their approach. In our economic system, the idea that 'more is better' has become so deeply embedded that it is now regarded as the only measure for success. If a learning moment does ever follow a harvest, it only serves to generate new initiatives that concentrate on bigger profits and even more new growth. No time is taken to consider the interests of the wider general good in the long term, such as social worth, ethics, ecology, sustainability, decent working conditions, etc. This results in the massive socio-economic and environmental damage that we see all around us today. We are paying a huge price for our obsession with growth without learning.

To make matters worse, this obsession also means that when moments of genuine crisis do occur, like the recent coronavirus epidemic, many companies are not prepared to respond quickly and effectively to the new situation. They have lost the habit of systematically and thoroughly reflecting on what they do. As a result, they do not have a back-up plan for when things go wrong, because their thinking is geared exclusively to growth scenarios. In consequence, many companies go to the wall, which simply serves to increase the level of social dislocation. The problem is further exacerbated by a similar approach from governments, who have also lost the habit of meaningful reflection, so that they far too often reach for old and outdated solutions to try and solve new problems.

It is also possible to see the same negative effects of an increasing focus on growth and profitability/productivity in the care sector. Short-sighted savings are made for purely financial reasons, without taking due account of important health and safety aspects or the need for preventative health care measures. Financial restrictions mean that more and more tasks need to be carried out by fewer and fewer people, so that the pressure of work is continually on the increase. In this kind of climate there is no room for calm reflection. At the level of individual care organisations, it is hard to see the direction that the care system in general wishes to take for the future, when the levels of available time and resources are constantly shrinking.

The results are not difficult to imagine. Medical, nursing and care staff are under non-stop stress, because they need to look after a growing number of people. As a result, patients and clients also scarcely find the calm and relaxation they need to reflect and learn. Because the caregivers are always so heavily burdened with work, there is little time and space for mental deepening, the development of willpower and the answering of questions like 'What do I want and what is the purpose of my life'. The chance to relax, reflect and enjoy good care, never mind re-energising your being, is becoming increasingly rare.

A similar pattern is evident in the private sphere. People who start a new relationship are often full of plans for how they wish to develop their future together: building their careers, buying a house, having children, etc. For the first five or six years, the relationship progresses smoothly, driven forwards by these high expectations and exciting new prospects. After this period, the couple can potentially harvest a number of benefits in various fields: domestic bliss, children, a healthy bank balance, successful jobs, a home that is bought and paid for.

Sadly, the partners all too often remain locked in the same routine, without pausing to reflect calmly on their original dreams and test them against their deepest wishes in the current phase of their life. Fundamental questions like 'Are we still on course?' and 'Is this what we really want?' remain unasked. As a result, they do not learn from what they have so far built up together and fail to initiate the reflection process that is necessary to develop new plans for the future phases of their relationship. Consequently, they fail to set new horizons for themselves. If they do undertake new initiatives, they tend to be little more than extensions of old initiatives: a bigger house, a second car, a better paid job. These are all variations of elements in their first growth cycle, but they lose their power to satisfy second time around. Because they neglect to take the necessary time for learning and reflection, many relationships find themselves breaking down through the sheer repetition of habits that have become meaningless.

All these examples illustrate the same problem that exists in so many domains of our modern society: the unwillingness or inability to learn and reflect. One of today's most popular mantras is: 'Standing still is moving backwards'. Whereas in reality, 'standing still' is precisely what we need, if we wish to re-energise and re-shape our lives in a deep and meaningful way. Instead, we focus on an endlessly repeated cycle of starting, growing and harvesting: launching new initiatives, cashing in our profits and achieving the highest possible profile, all of it accompanied by intense and not always healthy emotions, such as anger and greed. Consequently, we pay much less attention to kindness, concern and empathy for each other.

This has far-reaching implications for our society: too much shallowness and not enough deepening; too much superficiality and not enough meaning; too much short-termism and not enough reflection. As a result, we are never able to free ourselves from our old problems. Our inability to learn and reflect keeps us moving endlessly around in the same old circles, becoming increasingly exhausted and finally losing all sense of direction, bereft of the knowledge that comes from deep within about where we truly want to go.

Burnout

'This is how the entire course of life can be changed
– by doing nothing.'

Ian McEwan, On Chesil Beach

Burnout is also a symptom of the lack of learning and reflection that is so deeply ingrained in our society. People burn out because they repeatedly focus on growing and harvesting, always wishing to start with new initiatives without first taking the time to reflect. As a result, they are unable to draw lessons from their experiences to discover what it is that is making them feel so pressured.

By always taking on new tasks, by always expanding but never letting go, people eventually reach the limits of their endurance. Just as our breathing goes in and out, so following a period of personal expansion our connection with the world also needs to organically contract. Constantly expanding, growing and running blindly forward is a recipe for disaster.

In essence, burnout is a conflict situation. Most people see it as a conflict between themselves and an external agency: their employer, their colleagues, the amount of work they are expected to do, etc. But in most cases the conflict is actually with their own self. One part of them wants something; another part of them wants something different: 'I don't want that huge amount of work, but I do want the good salary that goes with it.' Or: 'I have often thought: "Stay at home, don't do this anymore". But I've got a mortgage to pay and the kids to put through university, so I have no choice.'

It is this field of tension that makes people ill. They externalise their illness by pointing the finger of blame at their work situation: 'My boss is a bully and he gives me far too much work.' But that is not usually the real cause of the problem.

By repeatedly focusing on action, expansion and results, the situation continues to escalate until the person reaches the end of their ability to cope and there seems to be no other solution than to stay at home. This is actually a symptom of mental narrowing. People stay at home supposedly to 'rest', but still spend most of their time worrying about their job and their social position. This kind of 'rest' will never result in a learning process. If, however, they can calmly reflect on the situation and take the time to stop and assess the things that are truly important to them, they can use the resulting inner strength to change things in their life in a manner that more truly connects with who they really are.

Shared Reading as a process of deepening

'A book must be the axe for the frozen sea within us.'

Franz Kafka

In our hectic, action-based and results-oriented society Shared Reading is like a welcome breath of fresh air. Simply the rhythm of someone reading aloud – which, once again, is six times slower than reading silently to yourself – forces people to slow down. This gives them a certain peace of mind, because it requires them to focus on something other than their daily trials and tribulations: and if they are concentrating on the text, they can't be worrying about something else. It is also brings them a kind of physical calm, since they need to sit still while they are listening, which prevents them from checking their smartphones or rushing off to their next 'urgent' appointment.

While experiencing this mental and physical calm, the text takes them down into the depths of human existence and their own being. Literary texts seldom deal with everyday banalities. By talking about the story or poem, people automatically find themselves at a deeper level of meaning that goes much further than a chat in the pub or on the train into work. In day-to-day life, this kind of conversation usually remains superficial, because it can sometimes feel uncomfortable to talk about serious subjects and you seldom know whether your conversation partner is willing to confront this discomfort. As a result, these conversations often leave you feeling frustrated, because you have not really been able to tell your story.

With Shared Reading, the subjects for discussion are, as it were, non-negotiable. The story or poem raises clear and serious themes that need to be addressed. The layered nature of the text quickly moves the participants' focus to a deeper level. If you are talking about an emotionally charged or philosophically coloured text, there is a much greater likelihood that it will stimulate you to talk about yourself, your experiences, your emotions and your thoughts. Such conversations are about something substantial and significant, something that looks beneath the surface. People can place their own experiences alongside those of the characters in the text, which brings calm and encourages openness. Even if they are talking about something deeply personal, the text continues to serve as a kind of buffer, so that the reactions of the other participants are not focused directly on the person in question. The conversation is always about the text – an imaginary world that makes connections with the real world of the readers.

The relaxation created by Shared Reading helps the participants to find inner calm, so that they can listen to what they are thinking and feeling. And because all different kinds of reflections and observations can be made without judgement, they gradually come to the realisation that they, as a person, are okay and that others are okay as well.

When the hurly-burly of the exterior world falls quiet and there is time to reflect, it is much easier to hear your own inner voice and to know how you should respond to it. This peace of mind helps you to see the direction you want to take in your life and encourages you, where necessary, to take the decisions that will make this possible.

In short, Shared Reading helps people to find their way to the essence of things. Conversations about stories and poems raise many different questions about human existence and its meaning. Why are we here? What do we want? Why do we do what we do? In the past, the answers to these questions were found in the religious sphere. That is no longer the case today, but we still have a need for answers in some shape or form. This is where literature can help. In literature we can find fragments of answers that sometimes complement each other and sometimes contradict each other, but they always offer us elements of meaning. One author writes with a sense of deep despair, while another writes with a sense of great exultation. But in the sum of all those different texts there is a kaleidoscope of perspectives that helps to shed light on the crucial 'why' questions. Stories and poems offer us depth, inspiration and dreams. They help us to connect with each other, to find new strength and to learn new lessons about ourselves and our lives.

'In the reading group we read *Silvano and Romildo*, a short story by Alberto Moravia. It is about two young adolescents who sell newspapers on the streets of one of Rome's more fashionable districts. You cannot tell for certain, but the writer suggests that they have been left to fend for themselves and are all alone in the world.

The story begins with the following words by Silvano: "I am not a cruel person. Quite the opposite. I am so good-natured and so gullible that everyone tries to take advantage of me, even those who don't really want to. And that is what Romildo did."

By talking about the story in the group, we discovered its deeper meaning. It is about people's eternal desire to have a friend and the price you are willing to pay to get one. We first discussed Silvano's fervour, uncertainty, generalisations and self-pity, but then we had deal with the crux of the story, its ultimate confrontation.

Romildo is cruel to Silvano; he even steals his girlfriend, Gesuina. One evening Silvano sees them kissing and cuddling in the twilight. Good-natured as he is, he goes and sits alongside them, saying nothing. Gesuina is furious and destroys him with the following words: "You're a coward, Silvano... Romildo is a thousand times more of a man than you'll ever be!" From that day on, Gesuina, Romildo and Silvano become inseparable.

One Saturday afternoon they make a trip to Ostia, on the banks of the River Tiber. Silvano feels cheerful and happy. He daydreams about making a voyage on the boat moored on the river bank. As usual, Gesuina and Romildo behave with cruelty and hostility towards him. Romildo challenges Silvano to kill someone as a proof of his friendship, although all he really wants is to have something new and interesting to tell his other friends. Gesuina plays the same game, but with much greater venom. Even the placid Silvano finally gives her a well-deserved slap across the face. As a result, the boys get into a fight, during which Romildo falls into the Tiber and is rescued by Silvano. But it changes nothing. "So it's agreed," says Romildo. "You commit the crime and I'll tell everyone about it."

An angry Silvano threatens Romildo with an oar and tells him to go. Later, Silvano gets into the boat and starts rowing. Suddenly, he realises that he is rowing upstream. He sees Romildo and Gesuina running along the river bank in the same direction and wants to catch them up, so that he can call to them to come aboard: "Then all three of us can enjoy the river together, like friends, as though nothing has happened..."

I have to admit that we didn't really understand the story, at least not at first. Why should you want to row after someone who always treats you badly, who wants you dead, and who keeps on wounding your soul, even after you have just saved his life? How could you possibly enjoy the river together, "like friends"?

The story eventually brought us back to our own project and our work on poverty. Isn't what Silvano experienced one of the keys to every human being, also for people in poverty? That after a long line of setbacks and after being lied to and cheated time and time again, you eventually reach a point where you no longer have the strength to see what talents you possess or to know who you really are and where you want to go? During the fragile transition from adolescence to adulthood, young people often go through a period of this kind, in which they search for ways to give meaning to their lives.

We would expect that anyone would want to rid themselves of bad friends, whether they are sadists or junkies, defeatists or materialists. Especially if you have a clear picture of what they are like and what they want to do to you. But sometimes we are just afraid of change. We prefer to hang on to what we have and who we know, rather than breaking with the past and facing the risks of a new world.

The nice thing about this story is that each of the three characters has such a searching moment. And of the three, it is actually Silvano who has the most spirit. He challenges himself repeatedly: "I am who I am and I cannot change". He observes and involves the outside world in his observations. But even if he is who he is and cannot change, this does not mean that he is unable to develop into a good person. Knowing yourself, being given opportunities and seizing those opportunities: the link with our work here is easily made. With the necessary support, the necessary confirmation and perhaps even with the same friends, you can become so much more.

This "standing still" is the best and most meaningful part of Shared Reading: the slow reading aloud, the slowing down of your thoughts, being on a journey together. But apart from getting to know and appreciate your fellow readers, reflecting

> and talking about the deeper meaning of the text is always an enriching experience.'
>
> Karim, reading companion for people in poverty

This greater deepening can be highly supportive for people in vulnerable positions. When the certainties in people's lives begin to crumble, reading literature together and talking about it can create opportunities for seeing more clearly what is truly important. This was also the experience of Hanne, a cancer patient who was read to in the final phase of her life by David, a medical student.

> When David was given the chance to read for a cancer patient in the hospital's oncology department, he immediately agreed. He is very interested in literature and as a medical student was keen to learn more about the human aspects of being ill.
>
> Right from the very first session, it was clear that Hanne, his reading partner, had a real feel for literature as well and could thoroughly enjoy listening to a good story. The conversations they had during the breaks in the reading were sincere and heartfelt, perhaps because Hanne had experienced many things in her life or perhaps because a few years of cancer treatment is likely to turn anyone into a wise philosopher.
>
> The trajectory foresaw ten reading moments. David and Hanne set the dates in their diaries on a weekly basis, falling neatly between Hanne's chemotherapy sessions. The nursing staff in the department soon got used to seeing David read to Hanne and discretely kept their distance during the subsequent discussions, so as not to disturb them. Hanne repeatedly told her doctor just how much she enjoyed the sessions and how much good they were doing her. "I think it's the same for David," she added with a

smile. True enough, everyone in the department could see that it was an intense process on both sides.

During the reading sessions David and Hanne were able to connect with each other in a warm and genuine manner. Hanne knew that her medical situation was not good and the stories gave her the opportunity to reflect on her life and to be grateful for what it had given her.

When a new course of therapy failed to have the desired effect, Hanne's condition quickly deteriorated. By the time the next reading session was due, it was clear that she was dying. No one was allowed into her room, with the exception of her husband and daughter. And David. He was the only non-family member who was permitted to visit Hanne to say goodbye. The collection of short stories from which they had been reading was still on her bedside table when she died...

Taking people seriously

Deepening is important, also for people whose mental and/or physical condition is fragile or who are in some way dependent on care. All too often, these people are no longer taken seriously, simply because they are seen as being too vulnerable or too old.

I know of one elderly lady who moved into a residential care centre because she was no longer physically able to live safely at home. She had been an avid reader since the days of her youth and literature had been a constant source of pleasure and enrichment in her life. In the care centre, however, she found herself expected to follow a fixed weekly programme, like all the other residents. Instead of amusing herself with Tolstoy or Murakami, she was now encouraged to play cards and take part in the weekly session of bingo. But she was no good at cards and hated bingo. She missed her literature.

When she mentioned this to the director of the care centre, he realised that his team perhaps needed to think about extending the range of available activities for the residents. Just because you are vulnerable, this does not mean that you have no further need of deepening. Just because you are old, this does not mean that you have answered all of life's questions. Even for patients and clients in a care context, literature can offer the crucial meaning and purpose for which we are all so desperately seeking.

'In our day-care centre, Shared Reading was something different. Most of the activities are based on doing something physical, but the reading group was typified above all by a sense of calm. True, this is not something for everyone, but for the people who took part it clearly had a beneficial effect on their personal life. Shared Reading is an activity that makes people think – and that is never a bad thing.

What struck me most was the way the participants in the reading group later repeated everything that had happened during their reading session to all the other people in the centre.

Before long, everyone knew what had been read and discussed: who the main characters were, what they had experienced, what they had decided... The story was passed on from person to person, almost as if it was a real event. In this way, the reading activity reached far more people than we had originally anticipated!'

Riet, director of a day-care centre for psychologically vulnerable people

Tips for practice

'Words are the mysterious passers of the soul.'

Victor Hugo

1. Don't rush things. Give the participants the necessary time to settle down and become fully engaged in the moment before you start reading.
2. Read the text at a comfortable, steady speed. Practice at home by reading the complete text out loud. This will help you to find the right rhythm and to identify the more difficult passages.
3. When you come to the end of a reading fragment, allow a few moments of silence before you ask your first question. Do not be afraid to allow similar moments of silence during the subsequent discussion of the text.
4. As the reading companion, always try to be fully present in the discussions that arise from the text. Try to exude a sense of calm, since this will make it easier for the participants to give space to their emotions and thoughts, before allowing them to sink in.
5. By allowing some of the participants to read aloud, you can give the opportunity to people who remain silent during the discussions to make themselves heard.
6. When the session is over, allow the participants a few moments to reset their focus on the outside world. Do not hurry them out of the door!

Epilogue

by Jane Davis

Dumb yearnings, hidden appetites, are ours,
And they must have their food.

> William Wordsworth, Fragment from:
> The Prelude, Book V – 'Books'

I first visited Belgium when I was invited to come and speak at a conference in Antwerp in 2012. Among the many enthusiastic people I met on that occasion was Dirk Terryn, who was to become, with Jan Raes and Erik Van Acker, one of the founders of Het Lezerscollectief. Dirk and his colleagues have remained committed and creative colleagues ever since, so it is a great pleasure to write this afterword for Jan's book, the first to be written about Shared Reading outside of England. *Shared Reading, The Ultimate Therapy* adds to the growing body of research into and practical guides about Shared Reading which have been developed by my husband Professor Philip Davis and my long standing Liverpool University colleague Professor Josie Billington. I hope it will be widely read by NHS, Social Care and other colleagues in the UK and beyond, especially those practising psychotherapeutic group work.

How Shared Reading came to be is a story I've told before but for any new readers: I was a reading child who had a tough childhood and went to many different schools, none of which I attended properly, and though I was a bright kid, my moving around and my absenteeism, and later, drug use, ensured I did not do well in the educational system. From the age of the twelve, I was often a runaway, but I always had books in my backpack – oddities and bestsellers like *Love Story* or *The Worm Oroborus*, for sure, but also great literary works like the plays of Samuel Becket and Shakespeare, the poems of Yevtushenko, and novels, *The Catcher in The Rye, A House for Mr Biswas, Crime and Punishment*. Books gave me models and examples, windows and escape hatches, and, despite having little or no education, I became an adult with a taste for serious reading.

Later, as a young single mother, I went to university to read literature. This was in the days of government grants for university students and after being a waitress and a barmaid, it seemed astonishing to me that I would be paid to read for three years. I couldn't help but notice, though, that there were not many people like me at University, and University literature did not want us to read as I did, as Charles Dickens says in *David Copperfield*, for life. These were the years of high theory in the world's university literature departments – all Lacan and Derrida and no sense of reading for one's personal self. Fortunately, at Liverpool University I eventually met my future husband Philip Davis and my teacher and PhD supervisor Brian Nellist: for both of them, there was no such thing as art for art's sake, it was always reading for life's sake. Phil, Brian and myself developed the 'for our sake' reading practice at Liverpool which had its best expression in Phil's two MA courses, first Victorian Literature and later, Reading in Practice. Meanwhile, for reasons to do with my personal biography and family, I left the university and began to develop the community reading practice that became Shared Reading, through the organisation I founded and have led for twenty years, The Reader.

All the elements Jan Raes describes here – warm and gentle welcome, personal connection, self-agency, a supportive and non-coercive group dynamic – were present from the first. And reading aloud? It was a practical response to the fact that some in my very early groups could not read. Reading aloud brought the text to life before us all, and meant that widely differentiating levels of formal education were evened out. From the early groups around the turn of the millennium, we grew to become a formally constituted organisation in 2008, when The Reader became the first Arts spin-out business from the University of Liverpool. Speaking about our work at the London Book Fair, I met Geert Van den Bossche, then of the Flemish Publishers organisation who said to me, 'We need this in Flanders – I'll arrange for you to come and speak' and so it was that I eventually met Dirk, Jan and Erik and we began our long established mutually valuable working partnership.

Initially, UK Shared Reading groups were run almost exclusively by our staff members. But we learned from Het Lezerscollectief that it would be possible to adapt our model, and train committed volunteers in partner organisations to develop groups. For us this has multiplied our reach and geographical spread tremendously. We now have the ambition to become a large scale movement, finding dedicated readers wherever they are and offering, through training and support, the means to develop Shared Reading. Our groups meet in libraries and community centres but also in Care Homes and Dementia Care Centres, our Reading Heroes programme pairs adult readers with individual children in foster care, and we work with those in rehab programmes or mental health services. We also work in nearly 40 secure settings, reading with people in prison or probation services. These latter groups are mostly staff-led, though we also train some prisoners and prison officers to run groups, too.

Over time, starting with Belgium and Denmark, Shared Reading gradually found partners in many countries around the world, from New Zealand to the USA, and with that in mind The Reader began to develop the idea of an International Centre for Shared Reading in about 2011. The idea was to find a building where we could build a model community held together by Shared Reading and host training for people in the UK and beyond. We opened Calderstones Mansion in September 2019 and welcomed visitors from Het Lezerscollectief soon afterwards. Due to the Covid-19 pandemic, many groups have had to move online, and have shown us that new areas of Shared Reading are now possible. During the extended lockdowns, we've run Shared Reading training online too, and it is terrific to see that things I'd have said were impossible ('we've got to be together in the room!') simply aren't true. Necessity and 'needs must' prove otherwise.

Het Lezerscollectief uses the same methodology as the one we at The Reader have developed over the last twenty years. For both The Reader and Het Lezerscollectief, Shared Reading is a common source of inspiration, connectedness and collaboration.

I look forward to seeing the impact of this book and the future developments that lie in store.

Jane Davis

The cycle of healing and integration

The cycle of starting, growing, harvesting, learning and relaxing that we have followed in this book is a highly stylised scenario. It is a model to indicate a process that in reality is much more active, in which the different phases run into each other and the movement can sometimes be backwards as well as forwards. Some people even bypass certain phases but still manage to reconnect with the next stage of the sequence. Nobody follows a perfectly linear trajectory in his or her thoughts and emotions. The road to our final destination always involves the occasional detour.

Nevertheless, this model is an interesting tool to demonstrate what happens to people during a session of Shared Reading. Taking the time to stand still with each other to examine a literary text sets in motion a process of healing that guides the participants through the entire cycle from starting to relaxing, sometime more than once during a single reading session. In each of these phases, the readers are offered the opportunity to achieve greater wholeness and integration in many different areas of their life.

Across the duration of a series of reading sessions the same dynamic is generated, in which people start full of expectation and curiosity, grow in terms of expanded insights, harvest the fruits of these insights, learn to let go of the things they no longer need, and calmly reflect on what this means for their life, before starting the cycle again.

Shared Reading is a highly valuable and efficient instrument for use in care settings. It is a process that is accessible for everyone, since it requires no training or background knowledge. This low threshold makes it possible for caregivers to guide their clients and patients with a minimum of fuss and delay through the beneficial Shared Reading process that offers numerous opportunities for growth and healing. People can enter the free space that Shared Reading creates, released from the burden of their medical history and/or prognosis, safe in the knowledge that no one will judge or evaluate them. They are there in all freedom. They listen, read and talk. From person to person, as equals. They can do as much as they wish, but are obliged to do nothing. This alone has an immense healing value and is far more effective than any formal therapy or course of medication. In this sense, Shared Reading is, if not the ultimate therapy, at least a highly rewarding and enriching therapy: a therapy that has no 'must' but leads people to healing and fulfilment simply through the freedom it offers.

Het Lezerscollectief

Het Lezerscollectief trains reading companions and organises Shared Reading sessions at a wide variety of different locations; for example, care institutions, schools, prisons, organisations helping to combat poverty, etc., but also at many other places where people just want to start a reading group. The reading companions are either members of staff of the organisation where the reading session takes place or else they are external volunteers. After completing their basic training, they undertake to read aloud for a group and occasionally follow further supplementary training.

Het Lezerscollectief is a learning network. In addition to basic training, we also provide the reading companions with the necessary tools and support to do their work with the reading groups. We make available collections of stories and there is an online platform with a library of texts suitable for being read aloud. We also organise intervision days, theme days and network days, where reading companions can exchange their experiences and get to know each other. Over the years, our relationship with The Reader has become ever closer. For example, our organisational model inspired The Reader to also start working with volunteers, while The Readers' ideas have been a constant source of new initiatives for us. Since 2020, Het Lezerscollectief for Belgium and The Netherlands has become an official partner of The Reader and the International Centre for Shared Reading in Liverpool. This was a fine confirmation of a warm and mutually inspiring collaboration.

Starting with Shared Reading?

Het Lezerscollectief organises a number of basic training courses each year for people interested in becoming reading companions. The course lasts for three days and immerses candidates in the Shared Reading methodology. First, you experience what it is like to be a participant, before gradually moving on step by step to learn in small groups what things are important in practice for the good supervision of a reading session.

Following this training, you can start working with reading groups. After roughly three months, there is a return day that gives you the opportunity to exchange ideas and talk about your experiences, as well as asking questions about issues you have encountered during these first early sessions.

The organisation for which you intend to read commits to pay for your training, to provide you with the necessary time and a suitable location in which the reading group can meet, and to make any other necessary practical arrangements. A volunteer is never expected to pay for his or her own training.

You can find more information about the basic and supplementary training of reading companions and about the organisation and activities of Het Lezerscollectief on our website, which also contains an inspirational interview with Jane and Phil Davis of The Reader.

lezerscollectief.be
lezerscollectief.be/de-ultieme-therapie

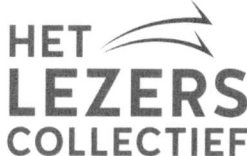

official partner of:

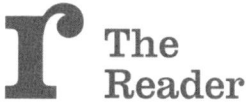

Sources for the literary fragments

Kader Abdolah, 'En toen waren wij aan de beurt', *De meisjes en de Partizanen*, De Geus, 1999 (translation by Ian Connerty, under permission of the author).

Lewis Carroll, *The Adventures of Alice in Wonderland*. Whitman, 1945.

Paulo Coelho, *The Alchemist*. Harper One, 1993 (translation by Alan R. Clarke).

Samuel Taylor Coleridge, 'The Rime of the Ancient Mariner. Text of 1834'. Retrieved from [https://www.poetryfoundation.org/poems/43997/the-rime-of-the-ancient-mariner-text-of-1834]

Charles Ducal, 'Judith', *De meesterknecht*, Atlas Contact, 1992 (translation by Ian Connerty, under permission of the author).

E.M. Forster, *Two cheers for democracy. Collection of essays.* Mariner Books, 1962.

William Ernest Henley, 'Invictus', 1888. Retrieved from [https://www.poetryfoundation.org/poems/51642/invictus]

George Moses Horton, 'On Liberty and Slavery', 1829. Retrieved from [https://www.poetryfoundation.org/poems/52307/on-liberty-and-slavery]

Ian McEwan, *On Chesil Beach*. Anchor Books, 2007.

Elif Shafak, TED Talk: *The politics of fiction*, 2010. Retrieved from: [www.ted.com/talks/elif_shafak_the_politics_of_fiction]

William Shakespeare, *Hamlet*. Retrieved from [http://shakespeare.mit.edu/hamlet/full.html]

Toon Tellegen, 'I drew a line...', *About Love and About Nothing Else*. Shoestring Press, 2008.

Maud Vanhauwaert, interview in: *Verbinden, verruimen, verdiepen. 25 jaar CANON Cultuurcel*. CANON, 2020 (translation by Ian Connerty).

Jeanette Winterson, *Why be happy if you could be normal?* Vintage, 2012.

William Wordsworth, Fragment from 'Book V – "Books"', *The Prelude*, 1850.

William Butler Yeats, 'The Lake Isle of Innisfree'. *Modern Poets* (edited by Jim Hunter), Faber Educational Books, 1968.

This book was originally published as *Samen Lezen.*
De ultieme therapie, LannooCampus, 2020.

D/2021/45/144 – ISBN 978 94 014 7664 5 – NUR 890, 770

COVER DESIGN Sarah Schrauwen
INTERIOR DESIGN LetterLust | Stefaan Verboven
EDITING OF ORIGINAL TEXT Mia Verstraete
LITERARY EXTRACTS ENGLISH EDITION Dirk Terryn
TRANSLATION Ian Connerty

© Jan Raes & Uitgeverij Lannoo nv, Tielt, 2021.

LannooCampus Publishers is a subsidiary of Lannoo Publishers,
the book and multimedia division of Lannoo Publishers nv.

All rights reserved.
No part of this publication may be reproduced
and/or made public, by means of printing,
photocopying, microfilm or any other means,
without the prior written permission of the publisher.

LannooCampus Publishers
Vaartkom 41 bus 01.02   P.O. Box 23202
3000 Leuven   1100 DS Amsterdam
Belgium   Netherlands
www.lannoocampus.be   www.lannoocampus.nl